fit
over forty

Sherri McMillan

fit
over forty

The winning way to lifetime fitness

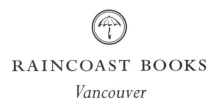

RAINCOAST BOOKS

Vancouver

Dedication

I dedicate this book to my husband, Alex, my gift from God.

Acknowledgements

As with any published work, there are numerous people who have provided support, feedback and guidance. They all deserve recognition.

I would like to express my extreme gratitude to the team at Raincoast Books. I appreciate the ongoing support you've given me. I'd like to offer a special thanks to my editor, Brian Scrivener, for working with me for a second time.

My thanks go out to my teachers and role models who have provided me with the knowledge, tools and experiences to present this material: Maureen Hagan, David Patchell-Evans, Daniel Kosich, Wayne Westcott, Len Kravitz, Allan Martin, Jack Taunton, Doug Clement, Ross Gurney and Peter and Kathie Davis. I would also like to thank IDEA, IHRSA, CanFitPro and other fitness conferences for their commitment to providing education to fitness leaders so we can do our job effectively and safely.

I'd also like to thank the *Province* newspaper, *Chatelaine* magazine and other trade journals and publications for giving me the opportunity to write and develop my skills.

I thank Nike and PowerBar for their continuous support and belief in my vision.

Thanks to the models; Brian Scrivener and Sandy Boucher. I also thank John Darch, our excellent photographer, and the Terminal City Club in Vancouver, British Columbia, for allowing us to use its beautiful facility as the location for our shoot.

Thanks to my friends and family who support me unconditionally in all my pursuits. I love all of you so much.

And last, but definitely most, I'd like to give thanks to God for His blessings.

Raincoast Books acknowledges the ongoing financial support of the Government
of Canada through The Canada Council for the Arts and the Book Publishing
Industry Development Program (BPIDP); and the Government of British
Columbia through the BC Arts Council.

Typeset by Jacqueline Verkley

NATIONAL LIBRARY OF CANADA CATALOGUING IN PUBLICATION DATA

McMillan, Sherri.
   Fit over forty

Includes index.
   ISBN 1-55192-386-6

1. Physical fitness. 2. Health. I. Title.
RA777.5.M35 2001   613.7′0446   C2001-910183-X

LIBRARY OF CONGRESS CATALOGUE NUMBER: 2002095543

Raincoast Books   *In the United States:*
9050 Shaughnessy Street   Publishers Group West
Vancouver, British Columbia   1700 Fourth Street
Canada   V6P 6E5   Berkeley, California
www.raincoast.com   94710

Printed and bound in Canada

10 9 8 7 6 5 4 3

Contents

Contents continued

Introduction

Imagine life the way you'd like it to be when you're 75 years old. Imagine that you're still able to participate in the recreational activities you enjoy — hiking, skiing, golf, tennis, camping, swimming, cycling and so on. Imagine that you're still able to travel the world, play with your grandkids, and are in no need of any assistance to perform daily chores and activities. The enjoyment and quality of your life is great. You are physically, mentally and spiritually fit and healthy. Life is good.

Now imagine the opposite scenario. Imagine you're 75 years old and you need a motorized wheelchair to get around. Imagine that you've been admitted to a nursing home because you can no longer take care of yourself. Imagine that you've become a burden to your children. Imagine that the relationship with your grandkids is superficial and strained because you're depressing and no fun to be around. Imagine that you never go outside because it's such a hassle. Imagine that every joint and muscle aches all day long. You can't get out of a chair on your own. You can't take a bath or go to the washroom on your own. Imagine a state of being in which you are physically, mentally and spiritually unhealthy. Wow, that's depressing!

The reality is that what you do today will determine the type of existence you can expect as you get older. Of course, there are accidents and genetic disorders, illnesses and diseases that may affect the quality of your life, but generally your health is a matter of choice, not chance. The lifestyle that you are living today will cause you to age more slowly or more quickly than your chronological age. It doesn't take a scientist or researcher to convince us that this is true. There are lots of examples of people who have always been healthy and fit and in their later years still have the energy and ability to enjoy life.

A company named FitnessAge, based in San Diego, California, has devised a formula to measure this phenomenon. What they call "FitnessAge" is a physiological assessment that scientifically calculates whether someone is aging more slowly or more quickly than average for his or her chronological age. The assessment involves tests that measure four components of fitness: cardiorespiratory, body composition, muscular strength and endurance and flexibility. At the conclusion of the test, the individual's results are plugged into a mathematical formula and compared with a database of 60,000 other results to determine the subject's FitnessAge.

Let's say that an individual is 40 years old but has never exercised and eats poorly. His FitnessAge may be that of a 60-–year–old. This means that he is aging more quickly than he should, due to his poor lifestyle. For a lot of people, finding this out may put things into perspective and will be the kick in the butt they need to start exercising and taking better care of themselves.

Most people realize that they should be exercising — everybody knows it's good for them. But most people don't exercise — they just *think* about starting an exercise program their entire life. There's a definite gap between knowing what we should be doing and actually doing it. Most people need a compelling reason, a motivating force to get started and stick with an exercise program. After someone receives a poor FitnessAge score or other fitness assessment from a medical or fitness professional, the common response is "Wow, I knew I was out of shape, but I didn't realize how out of shape I really am. I must do something about this." Often, this is when they lock into an exercise program.

In contrast, if an individual is 40 years old and has been working out regularly and taking good care of herself, she could have the FitnessAge of a 20–year–old. Imagine her response after getting that score. The common reaction is a big smile and a shout of "YES!" It is a definite ego booster. It's the pat on the back that she deserves. It's a reward for all her effort and discipline. It definitely reassures her that she has been doing the right thing and motivates her to keep on exercising and eating well.

I had the honor of meeting Jack La Lanne, the pioneer of fitness training in North America. He opened the first fitness club in the United States, he was the host of the first TV fitness show and he has been exercising every day since he was young. For decades he has been spreading the message regarding the importance and benefits of regular exercise, and he has become a living testament to why we should all be following in his footsteps. I met him when he was 85 years old. Imagine our common perception of the average 85-year-old — definitely frail. Well, Jack was not your typical 85-year-old man. He could still perform 20 full push-–ups on his fingers and toes, with perfect form. He still exercises every day and travels around the world with his wife, Elaine. Most people can't keep up with his energy and passion for life. He fills a room with laughter and has inspired thousands. And get this — his FitnessAge is that of a 29-year-old male. He's a great example of our ability to add years to our life and life to our years.

Let's face it, aging is an inevitable part of life. We're all aging by the second. But because of the huge population of baby boomers, this natural process will place an incredible strain upon our society. By the year 2021, approximately 16 per cent of our population will be above the age of 65. This will threaten our medical system, and even more staggering is the estimation that nearly half this population will have some degree of physical debility. As aging and a subsequent loss of strength occurs, it has an enormous effect on the capacity of individuals to lead viable and independent lives. This means an increase in hospitalization, nursing home placement and greater use of formal and informal home health care services. If it weren't for modern medical technology, many people would die at a much younger age. Instead, many unhealthy people are kept alive through medical advances and then endure a life full of pain and discomfort. Definitely not what I imagine for my later years!

We can expect certain changes, such as graying hair and wrinkled skin, to accompany aging. In fact, the cosmetics industry benefits from our attempts to reverse some of these changes. But the debilitating effects of aging are particularly noticeable in the musculoskeletal system (the bones, muscles, joints, ligaments, tendons and cartilage). However, luckily, many of the changes commonly attributed to the process of aging are a result of physical inactivity or disuse. The adage "use it or lose it" rings true. Muscle tissue, strength, bone density, cardiovascular fitness, energy levels and functional performance appear to be preserved through exercise. There seems to be no magic pill or drug that holds as much promise for sustained health as a lifetime program of physical exercise and good nutrition.

And a lot of us are taking notice. We can look to movie stars to find the most obvious examples of people who are fighting and winning against the aging process: Sophia Loren, Clint Eastwood, Paul Newman, Meg Ryan, Kevin Costner, Tina Turner, Goldie Hawn, Cher, Dick Clark, Sean Connery and many others. Most people who are aging slowly have taken on the attitude "I may be getting older, but I'm not dead yet!"

As a baby boomer, you are a member of the largest segment of our society, and the wealthiest and most health–conscious group. You've got the money to take good care of yourself and you recognize the value of doing so. Over the past few years there has been an 81 per cent increase in the number of people between the ages of 35 and 54 purchasing a gym membership, a 116 per cent increase in those between the ages of 55 and 64 and an 804 per cent increase in those over the age of 65 joining a fitness gym. More and more people in their middle years are realizing that sickness and disease are preventable, and that the quality of life they enjoy now and in the future is directly dependent on whether or not they exercise.

By reading this book you are already demonstrating that you take your health and fitness seriously, and have been or are ready to commit to an exercise and nutrition program. Through these pages you will learn many of the steps necessary to live longer and to still have the energy to do the things you do now or have always wanted to do.

Hippocrates said it best thousands of years ago: "Speaking generally, all parts of the body which have function, if used in moderation and exercised in labors to which each is accustomed, become thereby healthy and well developed, and age slowly, but if unused and left idle, they become liable to disease, defective in growth, and age quickly." A recent U.S. surgeon general restated Hippocrates' views by saying that a sedentary lifestyle is equivalent to and has the same health risk associated with smoking a pack of cigarettes a day.

My goal is to convince you that exercise and good nutrition are necessary and critical parts of your life, so that no matter what obstacles surface you will continue to take good care of yourself — now and on an ongoing basis.

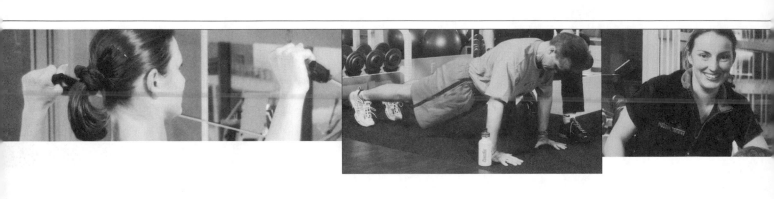

SECTION ONE the bad news

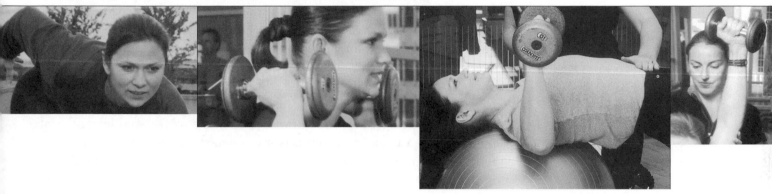

What will happen to us if we do not exercise? What types of changes can we expect to occur as we age and remain inactive? Let's take a look at the typical aging sedentary person.

Cardiovascular Fitness

For your car to work well, you have to run it regularly. Makes sense, doesn't it? Well, our bodies work in the same way. Our heart is a muscle just like any other muscle. If we condition our heart, it becomes a strong pump that, at rest, doesn't have to beat as quickly. For maybe 23 hours a day, seven days a week, our heart is beating more slowly and efficiently. An Olympics–level athlete can have a resting heart rate of 30 beats per minute.

But if we don't condition the heart, it becomes a weaker and less efficient pump. When a weak heart contracts it can generate only a small amount of force, so a minimal amount of oxygenated blood is pumped to all the tissues in the body. As a result, a weak heart has to pump more rapidly. A sedentary individual can have a resting heart rate of 80, 90 or 100 beats per minute. That's up to 70 more beats per minute than the heart of a highly trained athlete. Imagine any piece of equipment or machinery — if we have to use it more often, the chance for wear and tear and breakdown is greater. We can clearly see why people who are sedentary often experience more significant problems with their hearts.

If we remain sedentary, our aerobic capacity decreases at a rate of 10 per cent per decade after the age of 25. This means that we'll be huffing and puffing a lot more when engaging in any kind of physical activity. Household chores and other activities that we do every day will start to become more challenging, and in our older years will become maximal efforts. Consider the types of activities that are a maximal effort for you today — maybe an all-out sprint, or lifting a really heavy box or piece of furniture. If you remain sedentary, one day these types of activities will be impossible. A maximal effort in your later years will be trying to get out of your chair, climbing a set of stairs or carrying a bag of groceries.

You can imagine that if regular activities become extremely strenuous, most people start to avoid these movements to reduce fatigue. This creates a vicious cycle. Because of a sedentary lifestyle, an individual's aerobic fitness is reduced. This results in daily movements becoming very tiring. This causes the individual to avoid moving as much. This, in turn, negatively impacts on his or her aerobic fitness, so movement becomes even more exhausting and the person moves even less — and so on.

Muscle Tissue

Consider this: As we age we can expect to experience a 33 per cent reduction in muscle fibers over our lifetime. One–third of our muscle mass, gone! Women can experience an even more significant loss such that a sedentary woman, by the age of 80, will have only about a third of the muscle she had at 40. This equates to an average individual losing approximately three kilograms (seven pounds) of muscle each decade, with the loss accelerating after age 45.

It's interesting to note that this loss is dominated by a loss in the number and size of fast-twitch muscle fibers. These fibers are the ones responsible for allowing an individual to move quickly and to maintain agility, reaction time, strength and power. This is one of the major contributing factors causing older people to move very slowly. Watch as they get out of a chair, cross the street or try to make it across a room. It's not that they want to move that slowly. They physically cannot move any more quickly, due to the loss in these particular muscle fibers.

This loss of muscle mass significantly and negatively affects numerous other health factors and can lead to many complications. Read on.

"Our true age can be determined by the ways in which we allow ourselves to play..." — LOUIS WALSH

Metabolic Rate

Muscle tissue is energy-burning tissue. It is estimated that by adding about half a kilogram (one pound) of muscle to our body, we will burn an additional 30 to 40 calories per day. When we start to lose muscle, it negatively impacts our resting metabolic rate and we start to expend fewer calories every day. This means that, as we age, we can expect a two per cent reduction in metabolic rate each decade, with this loss paralleling the loss in muscle mass. This results in reduced caloric requirements — our bodies will need fewer calories per day. But since most of us have ingrained eating habits our diets are not adjusted and this can lead to creeping obesity, a phenomenon most aging adults experience.

Body Fat

Creeping obesity means we can expect to experience an average weight gain of 4.5 kilograms (10 pounds) per decade as we age into our seventies. We already discussed the fact that as we age we begin to lose muscle mass. So if we're losing muscle weight but gaining total body weight, where is all that extra weight coming from? You guessed it — body fat! The average woman's body fat as a proportion of her total body mass will increase from 25 per cent to 43 per cent as she ages, and a man's will increase from 18 per cent to 38 per cent. This increases the risk for obesity–related disorders such as hypertension, diabetes, osteoarthritis and coronary artery disease. Increased fatness triples the normal risk of heart disease and stroke.

Furthermore, body fat distribution changes as we age. More internal body fat, the fat that surrounds our organs, is deposited. That's a more dangerous type of fat deposit. And as estrogen levels drop, women typically start to store fat more like men, increasing their risks of heart disease. You probably won't be surprised to learn that 52 per cent of women in their fifties are overweight and more than a third of women aged 30 to 49 also weigh too much.

Strength

As you can imagine, a loss in muscle strength is a direct result of the loss in muscle mass that occurs as we age. At about the age of 50, strength starts to decrease so significantly that older adults in their seventies and eighties can expect to have only 50 per cent of the strength of young adults. This decline in strength is linked with increased risk of falls, increased frailty and loss of functional independence.

Bone Density

Bone density decreases at a rate of one per cent per year after the age of 35, so that eventually bone becomes brittle, porous and weak. For a woman, in the first five to 10 years after menopause annual bone loss increases to an average two per cent per year. Thus a woman can easily lose 25 to 30 per cent of her peak bone mass by age 60. This results in an increased risk of fractures to the forearms, lumbar area, wrists, vertebrae and hips. In fact, 25 per cent of post-menopausal women have enough bone loss to be diagnosed as osteoporotic. Experts suggest 25 million Americans have been affected by osteoporosis, with 80 per cent of these being women. You may be very surprised to learn that more women die each year from hip fractures related to osteoporosis than from breast cancer, uterine cancer and ovarian cancer combined. Each year about 300,000 people in the United States are admitted to hospital with hip fractures because of osteoporosis. Half of the victims never go home again, and one in five dies from complications within a year. These are alarming statistics.

Estrogen deficiency appears to be the most important cause of this bone loss. You should be aware that the risk factors for developing osteoporosis include being female, aging, family history of osteoporosis, inactivity, early menopause or hormone loss, poor diet or diet low in calcium, small/thin frame, abnormal absence of menstrual periods, anorexia nervosa or bulimia, smoking, excessive alcohol or caffeine intake, long periods of immobilization, use of certain medications (steroids, anticonvulsants, excessive thyroid hormones, certain cancer treatments) and, in men, low testosterone levels. Although women suffer from osteoporosis to a far greater extent than men

(5:2 female:male risk ratio), men are still susceptible. Of the five million American men suffering from low bone density, two million already have osteoporosis.

Changes in Posture & Gait

Do you have a relative who seems to get shorter every year? Well, this is not just your perception — it's a reality. We definitely get shorter as we age. We can expect to lose about 10 to 15 centimeters (four to six inches) in height by the time we reach our seventies and eighties. Postural deviations that cause slouching and fractures of the spine are the culprits. It is estimated that there are thousands of women with weak, porous bones who have compression and wedge fractures of the spine and aren't even aware of it. With each vertebral fracture, we lose approximately one centimeter (about half an inch) in height.

These changes, in combination with weak and tight musculature, lead to the typical *kyphotic* posture of older individuals — the hunched back posture. This results in a forward shoulder and head posture. Not very attractive!

We also change our gait, or walking posture. We position our feet in a wider stance to give us more stability. We shorten our walking stride to help maintain our balance. We are unable to lift our feet very high.

Loss of muscle mass also negatively affects our balance, so that older adults have a strong fear of falling. One in three adults over the age of 65 will fall at least once a year and 20 per cent of those aged 75 or older require medical treatment due to falls.

All our movements become slower and more cautious, due to poor balance and a fear of falling and hurting ourselves. We start to shuffle forward instead of walk. Add these changes to the fact that we may be taking medication and that our visual acuity may be reduced and you can see why there is an increase in falls as we age. Say goodbye to the spring in your step.

Loss in Functional Ability

Activities that we do every day, such as walking, climbing stairs, household chores, rising from chairs, carrying bags, shopping or taking public transit, become maximal efforts and exhausting and fatiguing movements. One study found that 76-year-old subjects couldn't negotiate a 50 centimeter (20–inch) step. Twenty-eight per cent of males and 76 per cent of females over the age of 74 in one study couldn't even lift 4.5 kilograms (10 pounds). Imagine how this affects our ability to carry our own groceries or lift our grandkids.

"Discipline is the ability to carry out a resolution long after the mood has left you. The mountain of soul-achievement and mastery of life cannot be scaled by the faint of heart. Without discipline, you won't make it to the mountaintop."

—Susan Smith Jones

Connective Tissue

As we get older, we experience a general loss of total body water weight. Approximately 60 per cent of our body weight is water, so you can imagine that as we start to lose water mass our tissues are not going to function optimally. Our connective tissue starts to become more rigid and inflexible, resulting in postural changes, increases in the chances of developing back and shoulder pain, and other injuries.

> "Age does not depend upon years, but upon temperament and health. Some men are born old, and some men grow so..."
>
> — TRYON EDWARDS

General Aches and Pains

With aging we experience degenerative changes in joint cartilage, causing more nagging aches and pains. Various forms of arthritis are the Number 1 source of pain and disability in the United States. The term "arthritis" covers more than 120 related diseases, including osteoarthritis, rheumatoid arthritis, fibromyalgia, bursitis, tendinitis and carpal tunnel syndrome. All of these cause pain and limited movement in the joints and related tissues. Bones, cartilage, synovial membranes, bursae, muscles, tendons or ligaments can all be involved.

The most common form of arthritis is osteoarthritis, also known as degenerative joint disease. It occurs customarily at the hips, knees and fingers and in the vertebral column. The next most common are rheumatoid arthritis, an autoimmune disease that is one of the most serious and disabling forms of arthritis, and fibromyalgia, a muscular disorder. All forms of arthritis limit our level of activity because of fatigue, pain and the fear of pain. These factors ultimately reduce the ability to walk, bathe, dress and perform household chores.

With age we also notice that our ability to bounce back after an injury is reduced. Remember when you were young and you could recover from an injury in no time? As we age, injuries occur more easily and are more difficult to treat.

Gastrointestinal Tract

There is a decrease in digestive secretions in the mouth, stomach, pancreas and intestines, which can reduce the ability of the mouth and the gastrointestinal tract to effectively digest and use carbohydrates, proteins, fats, vitamins and minerals. This makes it more difficult for us to obtain the nutrients we need to stay healthy.

We also know that as people age they begin taking multiple medications, which can negatively affect digestion and decrease appetite. For example, taking aspirin for arthritis can cause gastrointestinal bleeding; laxatives taken for constipation, if taken in excess, can interfere with absorption of fat-soluble vitamins or increase potassium excretion.

In addition, postural changes and tissue degeneration result in gastrointestinal disturbances such as bloating, cramping, gas and gastric acid (always embarrassing for anyone).

Hormonal Changes

As we age there are noticeable changes in our hormonal levels. A woman experiences drops in estrogen levels and men a drop in testosterone levels. You've probably heard more about the changes occurring in women. That's because the reduction in testosterone levels in men is more gradual and not as obvious.

Women start to notice their hormonal balance is off, demonstrated by heavier periods, longer periods, more closely spaced periods or perhaps bleeding during intercourse. This is usually a good sign that a woman is starting to experience the beginning stages of menopause, which usually occurs eight to 10 years before her last menstrual cycle. Generally, estrogen levels start to decrease between the ages of 35 and 40, with women noticing the symptoms between 42 and 47. The average age at menopause, defined as a loss of menstrual cycle for 12 months, is around 51. During this transitional stage, many women complain of hot flashes, problems sleeping, night sweats, depression, irritability, loss of concentration, weight gain and changes in fat distribution.

Emotional Changes

As we age, men and women often experience an emotional roller coaster.

Many of us are excited about getting to the age at which we'll be free of the kids. We look forward to having the time to travel and involve ourselves in recreational pursuits. Many women enjoy not having to endure the hassle of monthly periods, and others enjoy being able to have sex with their partners without concern about getting pregnant.

But then there are the down periods. We begin to recognize that our body is not looking and feeling as it did. We start to wonder where our 20-year-old shape went and realize that perhaps we've seen the last of our miniskirts and bikinis and muscle shirts.

Some of us start to contemplate death and question what's left of our lives. Others begin to search frantically for a higher meaning in life and grasp for a stronger, more spiritual foundation.

And then there's the midlife crisis many of us experience. It's a time for reflection and reassessment as we realize that time is slipping by. This leads some men to grasp for their youth one more time, attempting to achieve this through a new sports car or snappy clothing.

Many women are stereotyped as becoming more irritable and experiencing severe mood swings as they age. These developments may be related to sleep deprivation caused by hot flashes or to neurotransmitter changes associated with aging, or it may simply be that many women take a stand during this period. They may become more assertive — almost as if to say, for example, "I've given so much of my whole life to my family, and now it's time I stood up for myself. I deserve it!"

Sexual Patterns

Women experience some physiological changes that affect their sexual patterns. Their vaginal wall grows thinner and dries, and their natural lubricant is reduced. This can result in intercourse being painful. Many women have been found to experience a shorter orgasmic phase, making sexual intercourse less enjoyable.

While men are fertile into their eighth decade, it does take longer for them to achieve an erection as they age. On a positive note, they can keep their erection longer before ejaculation. But once they do ejaculate, their orgasm is less forceful and their resolution stage is longer — it takes them a bit longer to recover before being ready to go again. So for men there are some positives and some negatives with aging and their resulting sexual performance.

Pelvic Floor Dysfunction

Some of the changes in our pelvic floor functioning can be a real concern to a lot of people. As a woman's estrogen levels drop she is more likely to experience endurance incontinence, an extreme urgency to go to the bathroom and often not being able to make it in time. Stress incontinence, another dysfunction, causes a woman to lose urine when she coughs, laughs, sneezes, jumps or participates in high–impact classes or activities. This can be a result of a pubococcygeal muscle weakness and affects women more as they age because this muscle can be weakened by childbirth.

Changes in Senses

As we age, we experience definite changes in our vision, hearing and taste.

Many individuals complain of a loss of visual acuity that affects their ability to drive a car, recognize people, read, go to movies or play cards. Many experience a sensitivity to glare, while others will suffer from glaucoma, cataracts or macular degeneration.

There is less flexibility in the tissues inside our ears, making background noises more apparent and conversation more difficult to distinguish from background noise. This can be very frustrating; many struggle to hear what's being said and others become very sensitive to loud noise, even to the extent that loud sounds become painful to them.

We also experience changes in our taste buds, resulting in a decreased sensitivity to salt and sugar. Many older individuals increase the salt and sugar content in their diet in hope of improving the taste of food. When food can't be seen clearly or its aroma can't be enjoyed, often food starts to lose its appeal. Some people lose weight, due to a lack of appetite.

> "The greatest irritant to most people is not a lack of money or status, but ill health. Nothing shines brightly if we do not feel well…"
>
> — MARGARET STORTZ

Changes in Skin, Hair and Teeth

We don't need any scientific studies to know that we experience changes in our skin, hair and teeth.

Our skin loses its elasticity and becomes dry and wrinkly. Various types of spots form.

It's ironic, but as we age we start to lose hair where we once had it — on our heads — and grow it where we had none or at least less before — on our face, in our nose and ears and on our breasts. The texture of our hair changes, becoming more frail and thin, and our hair begins to lose its natural color and turn gray.

Our tooth enamel becomes thin and turns yellow, and gum disease is more prevalent. Chewing and swallowing will become more difficult.

Changes in Memory

Many studies indicate that as we age we notice a reduction in memory, even among those not suffering from Alzheimer's disease. People often comment that they require more time to process and recall information. "Where are the keys … the scissors …? Where is the cheque book?"

Changes in Sleep Patterns & Energy Levels

Many people say as they age that they have difficulty getting to sleep and frequently wake in the night. Many women suffer from disruptions to their sleep due to night sweats and hot flashes as they endure menopause.

Can you believe we're finally done? That was depressing, wasn't it? This section was intended to cause you to consider the consequences of living a sedentary lifestyle. If there isn't enough evidence here to persuade you to start or maintain a fitness program, I don't know what will.

" ...what a disgrace it is for a man to grow old without ever seeing the beauty and strength of which his body is capable."

— SOCRATES

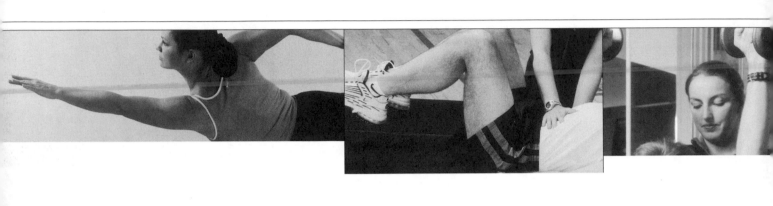

SECTION TWO the good news

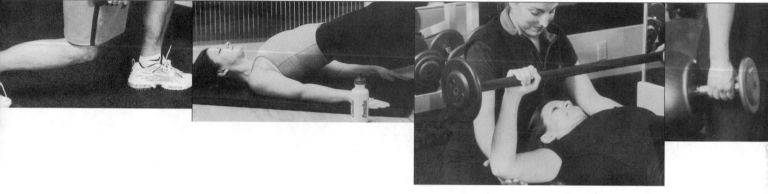

Here's the good news: Most of the age–associated changes we've just discussed can be prevented, reduced in severity or managed by participating in a regular health and exercise program.

The science is conclusive. Exercise and good nutrition are critical to our well–being, today and in our later years. We don't have to settle for "getting old" as we get old. Many are graciously fighting the aging process and winning.

Let's find out what you can do about it! Follow along with my Top 10 strategies for fighting the aging process for baby boomers.

Muscle Endurance & Strength Training

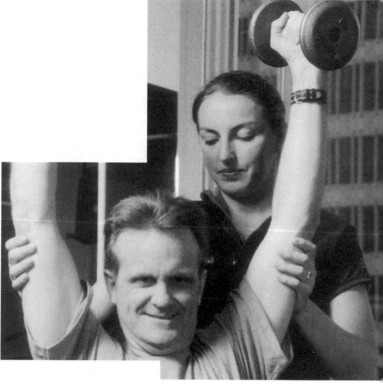

Many physiologists and researchers deem muscle conditioning to be the true fountain of youth — the "magic pill" to reverse or prevent a significant portion of the aging process. A good number of the changes people experience as they age are due to a loss of muscle mass. If we can maintain a significant amount of muscle tissue, we can expect to age much more slowly. Research indicates that general strength training can achieve the following results.

- Strength increased by up to 226.7 per cent. — that's a huge boost!

- Lean tissue weight increased by 1.3 kilograms (about 3 pounds) after eight weeks of strength training. Now remember it's estimated that each half kilo of muscle you have on your body will burn an additional 30 to 40 calories every day. This definitely raises your metabolic rate — in fact, by seven per cent. If you gain 1.5 to two kilos of muscle, you'll be burning 90 to 160 extra calories every day just by having more muscle on your body. This makes it so much easier to maintain your body weight and keep your body fat levels at a minimum.

- Lose 4 pounds of fat weight after three months of strength exercise, while eating 15 per cent more calories.

- Increased bone mineral density after four months of strength exercise (important for reducing risk of osteoporosis. It has been found that women over the age of 40 who engage in strength training not only don't lose bone mass but actually experience a one per cent gain in bone mass).

- Improved posture (most postural problems can be treated by following a structured muscle–conditioning program).

- Glucose uptake increased by 23 per cent after four months of strength exercise (important for reducing risk of developing diabetes).

- Gastrointestinal transit time increased by 56 per cent after three months of strength exercise (important for reducing risk of colon cancer).

- Reduced blood pressure after two months of strength exercise.

- Improved blood lipid levels after strength training (important for those with high cholesterol).

- Reduced low–back pain after 10 weeks of specific strength exercise.

- Reduced arthritic pain after strength training. (One study reported a 59 per cent decrease in joint pain.)

- Walking speed increased by 48 per cent, climbing power increased by 28 per cent.

- Decreased risk of falling. A study of women over the age of 40 found that the sedentary subjects experienced an eight per cent decline in balance, while those who practiced strength training demonstrated a 14 per cent improvement.

On top of all these benefits, muscle looks good, and it improves our posture so that we carry ourselves better and with more confidence. We move differently, with greater coordination and agility, and our performance in recreational pursuits is enhanced significantly.

Let's look at some research conducted on aging subjects.

Dr. W. R. Frontera performed a strength–training study on 60 to 70–year–olds. He had his subjects exercise at 80 per cent of their capacity, a pretty high–intensity program. The findings shattered myths about aging. There were no injuries and no cardiac episodes during the training protocol. In just 12 weeks, the muscles that were trained became 10 to 12 per cent larger and 100 to 175 per cent stronger! Traditionally, seniors have been advised to do strength–training exercise at only 40 to 50 per cent of their capacity — a much lower intensity — for fear of injury or other health risks.

Dr. Frontera's study showed that it's never too late to start, and it's okay to work hard at an older age because we will experience significant improvements at the higher intensity level. This type of increase in muscle mass and strength significantly improves an individual's body composition, posture, bone density, agility, coordination, power, reaction time and ability to perform daily movements.

Dr. Maria Fiatarone, another leading researcher for the Human Nutrition Center on Aging at Tufts University in Boston, performed·a study with high–risk subjects between the ages of 86 and 96. Each had at least two chronic diseases, including heart disease, diabetes or osteoporosis. Most relied on walkers or canes and several had leg muscles so weak that these people couldn't even rise from a chair without using their arms. The subjects exercised three times a week for eight weeks. In just eight weeks these frail, elderly men and women increased their strength by an average of 175 per cent. In a test of walking, speed and balance, their scores rose by an average of 48 per cent. Two participants discarded their canes. Imagine their improved quality of life. For this group, exercise is not about looking better — it's about living life to its fullest. If they can experience such dramatic improvements, just imagine the benefits you could achieve!

Another group of investigators at the University of Colorado compared sedentary and active postmenopausal women aged 50 to 72 with women aged 21 to 35. The older women who were not exercising showed the expected decrease in basal metabolic rate compared with the younger participants, but the older women who were physically active had the same basal metabolic rate on average as active women half their age. This means that active postmenopausal women will be much more able to maintain a healthy body weight as they age. So you have to question whether the common 4.5 kilogram (10 pound) weight gain every 10 years is a result of aging or just inactivity and a loss of muscle mass.

It's pretty clear that muscle endurance and strength training will bring forth numerous benefits. I'm sure you'll agree that it really does deserve the title "fountain of youth."

"Knowing is not enough; we must apply! Waiting is not enough; we must do."

JOHANN W. GOETHE

A Prescription for Muscle Endurance & Strength Training

Now here's the better news. You don't have to spend hours in the weight room seven days a week to experience these positive changes.

The American College of Sports Medicine recommends one set of eight to 12 repetitions (10 to 15 reps if you are 50 or older) for all larger muscle groups twice a week. The repetition zone between eight and 12 is the favored prescription because it will evoke improvements in both muscular strength and endurance. And can you believe that all you have to do is one set? Yes! No more two or three sets of the same exercise. For what we're hoping to achieve, all we need to do is one set of a variety of exercises. Of course, if you have more aggressive goals it may be necessary to perform multiple sets of each exercise, but for the majority of people one set is enough.

With this prescription, you need only spend about 30 to 40 minutes in the weight room twice a week. I hope you see the value of investing this small amount of time in your overall health.

Muscle Endurance & Strength Training Guidelines

A resistance–training program that does not focus on technique will get you results much more slowly and may put you at risk of injury. Here are some very important technique tips.

- Quality and execution of movement is critical. It makes no sense to perform 20 sloppy reps. It is far better to perform eight reps with perfect form and then take a break.

- Take it slowly. Proper resistance training is not a fast sport. Wayne Westcott, a leading strength and conditioning researcher, has determined that one repetition should take approximately five to six seconds; that is, two seconds to lift the weight and four seconds to slowly lower it in a controlled fashion. Most people lift much too quickly, using momentum instead of muscle. A proper set of 8 to 12 repetitions should take approximately one minute to complete. Proper execution of each rep is the most critical factor in weight training. Reps performed with poor technique will get you nowhere!

- Breathe. A proper breathing rhythm will make each set more effective. Focus on exhaling as you lift the weight or when you exert, and inhaling as you recover or lower the weight.

- Maintain good posture. Proper posture is critical to ensure you are working the correct muscle groups and not putting your body at risk of injury. If seated, sit up straight. Always keep your abdominals contracted through the entire set of any exercise. Pull them up and in toward your spine to help stabilize your trunk. Keep your shoulders back and chest lifted up and out during any seated, bent–over or standing exercise.

- A good exercise set will finish once you hit momentary muscle fatigue. This is the point at which you absolutely cannot do another rep with perfect form. If your set is supposed to be 8 to 12 reps but you can perform 12 to 15 reps or even more, you should perform the extra reps to hit momentary muscle fatigue, and next time increase the weight so that you hit momentary muscle fatigue within the suggested repetition zone of 8 to 12 reps.

- If you cannot perform 8 reps, the weight is too heavy. If you can perform 12 reps with perfect technique, increase the weight by five per cent.

- Never go to failure. Failure is when you continue the set with poor technique, or when other muscle groups kick in to help finish the set. It is important that you always avoid bad technique and muscle substitution.

HERE ARE DEFINITIONS TO CLARIFY THIS COMPONENT OF YOUR PROGRAM:

Repetition, or **rep**, refers to the number of times you perform an exercise without stopping. For example, 10 repetitions means you do that exercise 10 times.

Set refers to the number of times you perform a complete series of repetitions. For example, you may perform two sets of 10 reps.

- Perform your muscle–conditioning sessions on alternating days. Your muscles require a day of rest in between muscle–conditioning workouts.

- Put your mind into it. It is okay to let your mind wander while you perform some fitness activities. For example, you can jump onto a treadmill and plug in a seven–minute–mile pace and whether you think about it or not you will expend the same amount of calories. However, this is not the case with muscle–conditioning exercise. You must focus on what you're doing because there is such a strong connection between the brain, the nerves and the muscles. Studies show that if you concentrate on what you are doing you can significantly increase the amount of muscle activity measured during these exercises. So put down your magazines, cease all conversation and really focus on each set. Each repetition and each set will become much more effective and you will experience results much more quickly.

Which exercises will do the trick?

There are literally hundreds of different exercises you could perform to get the results you are seeking. Here are a few guidelines to follow when designing your resistance–training program.

Start with basic exercises. It is necessary to progress from exercises that require the least amount of skill, coordination, balance and overall fitness to exercises that maximally challenge these skills. This means that, in the beginning, very basic exercises will do the trick. As you improve and master the techniques, you should advance the program by incorporating more challenging exercises.

For example, when performing a chest press you might start on a machine that has a back support, so that all you have to think about is pushing the bar. As you master this skill and your muscle conditioning improves, you can try performing the exercise with hand–weights instead. Now you have to think about balancing the hand–weights, which adds a new dimension to the movement. Once you have mastered this skill you can progress to performing the exercise while lying over an exercise ball, instead of on a bench. Not only do you now have to think about the hand–weights, you also have to consider that you are lying on a moveable object, which will add a further challenge to the exercise.

You can follow this type of progression for any exercise. Every four to eight weeks, try to add a new challenge to any exercise that you are performing. But it is always important that you follow the appropriate gradual progression. You definitely do not want to attempt more challenging exercises without having first developed the basic foundation for the skill.

Change your program regularly. The only perfect resistance program is one that changes. A program that we design today may be perfect today, but in about four to eight weeks it will no longer be perfect and may be quite ineffective. This is due to the overload principle — a training principle to which all personal trainers must adhere in order to help their clients experience ongoing improvements.

When you first begin exercising, the body is exposed to a stimulus that it's not used to, and it will be forced to respond in a positive fashion by getting stronger and fitter. This is called a physical adaptation, which means that your body has structurally, biomechanically and physiologically improved. But simultaneous with the physical adaptation is the physical plateau that many people experience. To achieve ongoing results, the body must be stressed or stimulated to a greater degree than usual. We know that the body needs to be challenged in order to progress.

You can adhere to this overload principle by changing your program in a variety of ways. You can change the resistance you lift, the exercises you perform, the order in which you perform them, the number of sets or reps, the amount of recovery time you take between exercises or the number of days you work out each week.

This is where an investment in a personal trainer may save you a lot of time. It is not necessary for you to spend a fortune to benefit from his or her expertise. Even one or two sessions every two months, to give you advice about the changes required for continued results, will go a long way toward maximizing your workout time. You don't need to purchase a gym membership — many personal trainers will come to you and design a home program that you can follow. IDEA, an international health and fitness organization, released a statistic recently at one of its conferences. It said that only 25 per cent of people working out in a gym were getting the results they wanted, but 90 per cent of those achievers were working with a personal trainer. It is quite clear that having a personal coach to look after your progress and update your program regularly is an investment in your health worth making.

Choose functional exercises. You must ensure that you include functional exercises in your program. "Functional" means that the benefits you obtain from your fitness program will enable you to perform your day–to–day activities more easily and without getting fatigued, and allow you to participate in recreational pursuits with improved performance. This means that you should include exercises that are:

Although it is important to regularly overload the body, there is a fine line between overloading and overtraining, and it's important that you know the difference. Overtraining is when you have done more than your body is capable of handling. If you are overtraining, you may experience some of the following symptoms: ongoing and/or extreme muscle soreness; continual decrease in normal workout performance; persistent colds, headaches, injuries or other illnesses; loss of appetite; intestinal problems; loss of lean tissue; ongoing fatigue; changes in mood or attitude; unexplained losses in body weight; and/or cessation of menstrual cycle. If you are experiencing any of the above symptoms and cannot explain why, you should discontinue or reduce the intensity and volume of your training and visit a sports physician.

1. **COMPOUND.** A compound movement is one that involves many joints and muscle groups within one exercise. For the lower body, exercises such as lunges and squats are compound movements. For the upper body, exercises such as chin–ups and push–ups are compound movements. These types of movements are important because they train the body in a fashion that is similar to how we actually move in everyday life. For example, every time you get out of a chair, that's a squat. Every time you bend down to pick up something, that's a lunge. However, you should progress into lunges and squats in a gradual fashion. Start with mini–bends and progress into the deeper lunges and squats once you learn proper knee tracking and alignment and your muscles get strong enough to handle the deeper load. Many exercises in the weight room are unijointed and involve only one muscle area which is not really how our bodies move. Most of the movements we perform every day are compound. If we want to get stronger and be able to use this strength in our everyday lives, we have to train the muscles in a way that will allow those benefits to carry over.

2. **COMBINATION TRAINING.** These types of exercises are definitely compound in nature and involve combining two or more exercises into one complex, fully integrated, functional movement. For example, a squat with an overhead shoulder press is a form of combination training. A bicep curl while standing on one leg is a form of combination training. The theory behind combination training is as follows: Most movements that we perform every day involve the upper body having to work with the lower body; we have to balance our body and stabilize our torso. But most of the exercises we perform in the weight room isolate only one muscle group. So when someone is placed in an environment where the body has to use various muscle groups, the muscles don't know how to respond correctly and effectively because they've never been trained to do this. It would be similar to a football coach training each player independently. Although the coach could feasibly get each player into the best physical shape of his life, if that team doesn't get together and scrimmage the first game will be a disaster. Our muscles work in a similar fashion. That is, each can be strong independently of the others, but if they haven't learned how to react, oppose and resist each other the strength in the weight room will not carry over into the real world. There are many cases of people and athletes who are very fit in the weight room — that is, they can lift a lot of weight. But they go home and lift some furniture or carry heavy boxes and hurt their back and strain connective tissue because they haven't taught the muscles to work together. The message is this — you need to be strong in and out of the weight room. Combination–training movements will help you achieve this goal.

    Before I provide you with some practical exercise ideas, I want to make one point to my female readers. Many of you may be concerned about putting on too much muscle. I realize that most of you do not want to gain a lot of muscle or look like the women on the cover of *Muscle and Fitness* magazine. I assure you that you do not need to be concerned. Most women just do not have the natural levels of growth hormone and testosterone to develop muscles in this manner. Very muscled women are a very, very small per centage of our population and most of them work out for hours in the gym. Most are probably using some form of supplementation or ergogenic aid to help them achieve this type of build. Honestly, following these muscle endurance and strength prescriptions is not at all about getting bulky — it is all about keeping the muscle you've got!

> "Believe you can and you can. Believe you will and you will. See yourself achieving, and you will achieve."
>
> — GARDNER HUNTING

Muscle Endurance & Strength Exercise Program

Here is a sample program you can do in the gym. Notice that I alternate exercises between the upper and lower body, so that while the lower body is working the upper body gets a chance to recover and vice versa. Perform one set of each of the exercises. Remember to adjust this program. Don't get caught doing the same program months later. Make small changes each workout by increasing reps or resistance. Every six to eight weeks, see a trainer to make some more dramatic changes by including new exercises and altering the sequence.

COMPOUND EXERCISES

○ Assisted Chin-Up

UPPER BODY

WORKS THE LATS, BICEPS, FOREARMS

Assisted chin–up apparatus are very user–friendly and effective machines for challenging your upper body. The model at your gym may be either a stand–up or kneeling model, and it may be computerized or involve only a weight stack. The instructions on the front of the machine will clearly demonstrate how to complete the setup process. You will also notice that the chin–up exercise allows you to choose three or four different grips — a wide grip, a midgrip, a narrow grip or a reverse mid–grip.

Try all the grips to challenge your muscles with a slightly different stimulus with each set. Once you have decided upon the grip, technique is pretty simple. As you pull with your arms, your body will lift. Stop once your chin has cleared the bar. Slowly return to the starting position. Fully extend your arms without locking out your elbows. Try to focus on pulling with the muscles in your back rather than your arms. Perform a set of 8 to 12 reps (10 to 15 if you're 50 or older). This is a compound movement.

In the confrontation between the stream and the rock, the stream always wins — not through strength but by perserverance.

— H. JACKSON BROWN

○ Dumbbell Squat

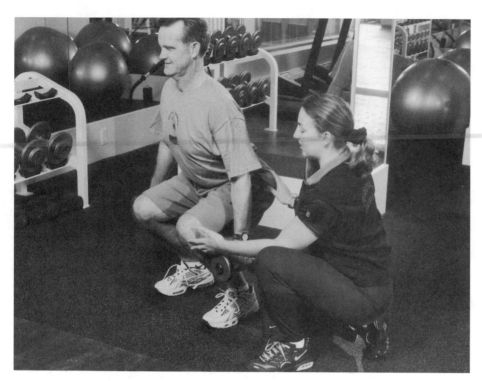

LOWER BODY

WORKS THE QUADRICEPS, HAMSTRINGS, GLUTES

The squat is a very effective exercise for the lower body. Start by standing with your feet apart, between hip and shoulder width. Hold a set of hand–weights at your side. Set your posture by contracting your abdominal muscles, pressing your chest out and up and your shoulders back and down. Start by slowly squatting backwards while keeping your kneecaps pointing forward — avoid allowing your knees to collapse inward. Try to keep your weight equally distributed on all four corners of your feet; avoid allowing your arches to collapse inward. Lower until your upper thighs are parallel to the floor; if you're just getting started with leg training or you feel any type of discomfort around your knees, perform only a mini–squat (don't go as deep). You'll notice that your upper body will come forward slightly while your buttocks travel backwards. Now slowly extend upward. If you're starting with mini–squats, focus on mastering your technique and drop lower and lower once your muscles get stronger. Perform a set of 8 to 12 or 10 to 15 reps. This is a compound movement.

Chest Press with Inner Thigh Squeezes

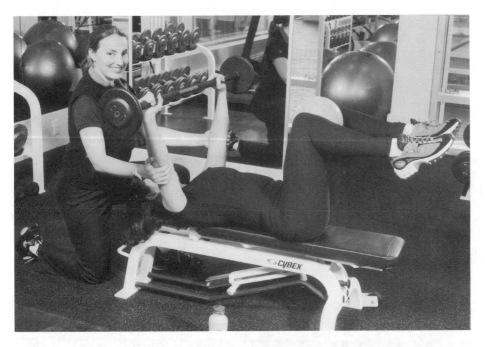

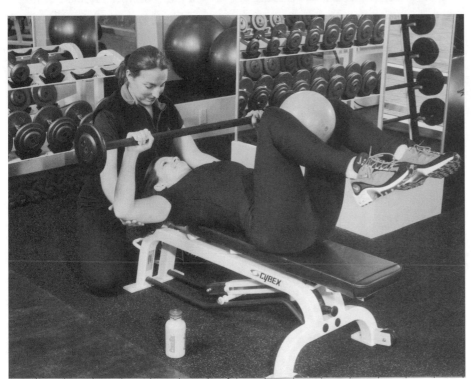

UPPER BODY

WORKS THE PECTORALS, TRICEPS, ANTERIOR DELTOID AND INNER THIGH MUSCLES

Lie back on a bench. Position your body so that your feet are suspended in the air (this will involve more balance and torso stabilization) and hold a ball between your thighs. Grab the barbell (you can also use hand–weights) a little wider than shoulder width. Lift the barbell off the rack and start with it positioned over your shoulders. Slowly, controlling the weight, lower the barbell toward the middle of your chest. Do not allow your elbows to drop below your shoulder joint — lowering below this point will place excessive stress on your shoulders. Now push your arms back to the starting position without locking your elbows. Make sure your abdominals remain contracted throughout the exercise. Perform a set of 8 to 12 or 10 to 15 reps. This is a compound movement.

⊙ Seated Hamstring Curl

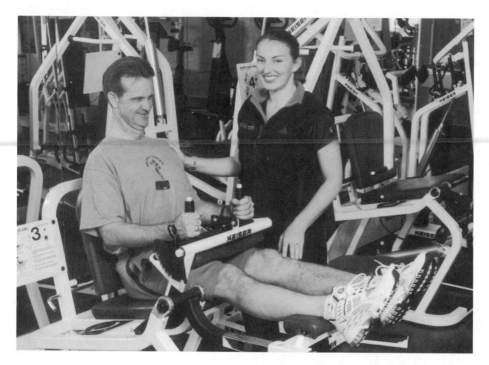

LOWER BODY

WORKS THE HAMSTRINGS

Most of these machines are adjustable to ensure proper setup for people of varying body proportions. Choose a seat setting that allows you to be in a position where your knees line up with the center of the pulley or the rotationary axis on the machine. This means that the machine will rotate along the same axis as your knee. You should be able to draw a straight line from the middle of your knee to the middle of the rotating point on the machine. Once you've positioned your seat correctly, you can adjust the upper pad onto your thighs so they are comfortably locked into place. Start by contracting your abdominals and stabilizing your torso and pelvis. Then slowly curl your lower legs toward your buttocks. Once you've hit the end range of motion, you can slowly release to the starting position while avoiding hyperextending your knees. Perform a set of 8 to 12 or 10 to 15 reps.

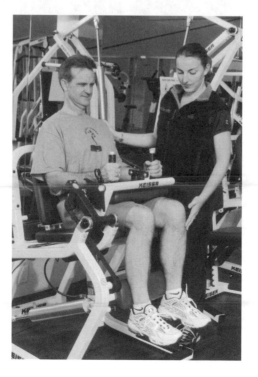

○ Seated Row

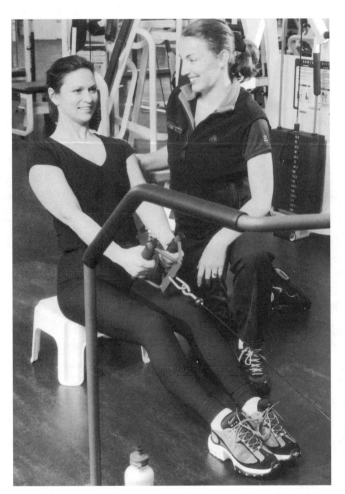

UPPER BODY

WORKS THE LATS, RHOMBOIDS, BICEPS, FOREARMS

Start in a seated position, knees slightly bent, abdominals contracted, shoulders back and down, chest lifted up and out, upper torso at a 90–degree angle. Your back is completely vertical. Pull the handle to your midsection. Keep the handles low and your elbows at your side, and avoid pulling your shoulders upward. Return slowly to the starting position, avoiding rounding your shoulders forward. Perform a set of 8 to 12 or 10 to 15 reps. This is a compound movement.

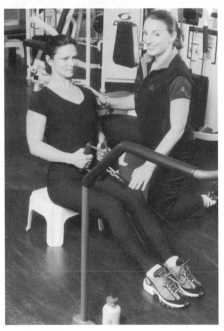

○ Lunge

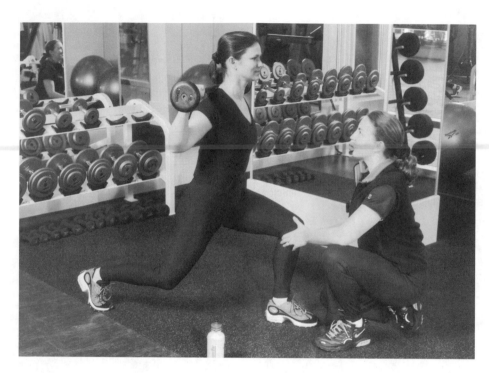

LOWER BODY

WORKS THE QUADRICEPS, GLUTES, HAMSTRINGS

Comfortably position a barbell on your shoulders or holding hand–weights. Stand with one leg positioned in front of the other. Keep the front knee over the top of the ankle. Keep the back knee underneath or slightly behind your hips. Slowly lower the back knee toward the ground, keeping the front knee over the ankle. The lowest point should be when your front knee is at a 90–degree angle or your upper thigh is parallel to the ground — only go as low as feels comfortable. Keep your body weight positioned over the front leg; this is your working leg. Maintain upright posture and keep your abdominals contracted. Remember, you can begin with just mini–lunges. Perform a set of 8 to 12 or 10 to 15 reps for each leg. This is a compound movement.

⊙ Push-Up

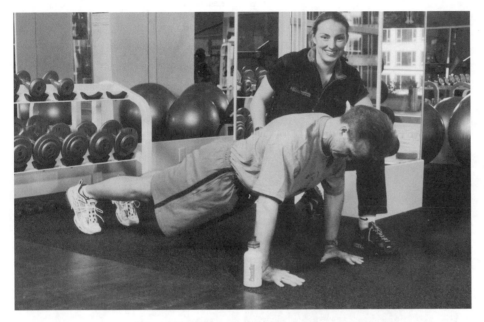

UPPER BODY

WORKS THE PECTORALS, ANTERIOR DELTOID AND TRICEPS

Lie on your stomach. Position your hands on the floor a few inches from your shoulder. Make sure your elbows are directly above or to the inside of your wrists. Bring your heels close to your buttocks. Keep your abdominals contracted and your back in its neutral position. Now slowly push up and slowly lower down to the starting position. Perform a set of 8 to 12 or 10 to 15 reps. As you advance, perform the same exercise from your toes. This is a compound movement.

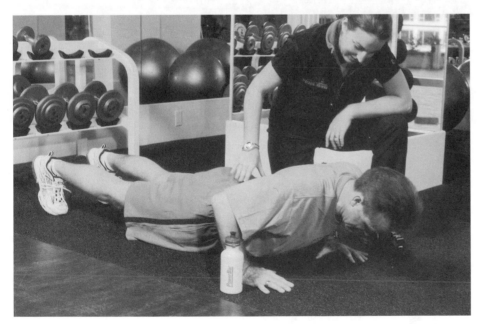

○ Step–Up

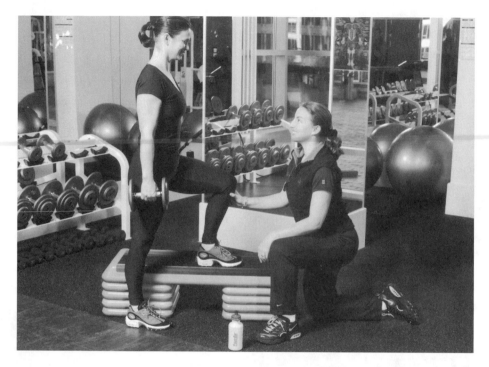

LOWER BODY

WORKS THE QUADRICEPS, GLUTES, HAMSTRINGS

Place a barbell on your shoulders or hold hand–weights. Position yourself in front of a bench or staircase, with one foot on the bottom or second step. Keep your kneecap facing forward and your weight distributed on all four corners of your front foot. Slowly step up, extending the supporting knee into a fully upright, balanced position. Now slowly lower yourself to the starting position. Perform a set of 8 to 12 or 10 to 15 reps for each leg. This is a compound movement.

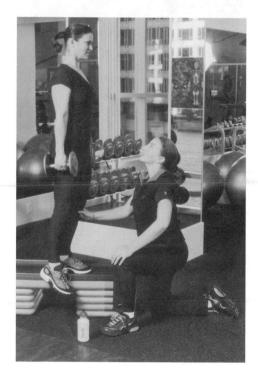

○ Lat Press–Down

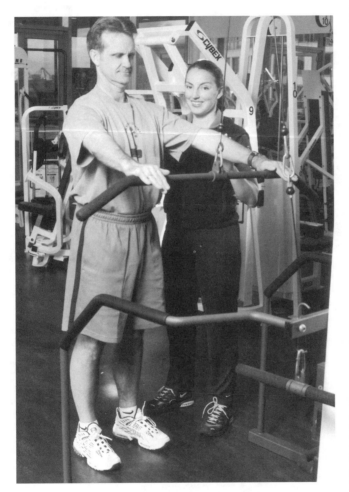

UPPER BODY

WORKS THE LATS

You can perform this exercise using a lat–pull–down bar, a T–bar or even an exercise tube. Start with both hands pressing down on the bar, with the arms extended straight out in front at the height of the shoulder. Keeping your abdominals contracted, torso stable and vertical, shoulders back and chest lifted up and out, slowly press the bar down toward your thighs. Slowly return to the starting position. Perform a set of 8 to 12 or 10 to 15 reps.

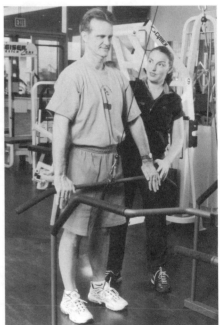

⦿ Prone Hamstring Curl

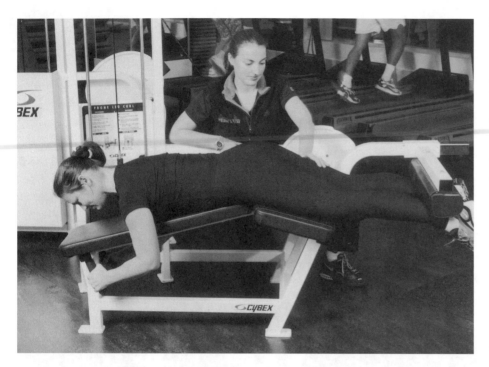

LOWER BODY

WORKS THE HAMSTRINGS

Position your body so that, while lying on your stomach, your knees fall just below the edge of the pad. This should position your knees so that the center of the point where the machine rotates lines up with the center of your knees. Adjust the ankle pads so that they rest just above your heels. Begin slowly to curl your lower legs toward your buttocks. Keep your abdominals contracted and your pelvis pressed firmly into the machine. Slowly release to the starting position, being careful not to hyperextend your knees. Perform a set of 8 to 12 or 10 to 15 reps.

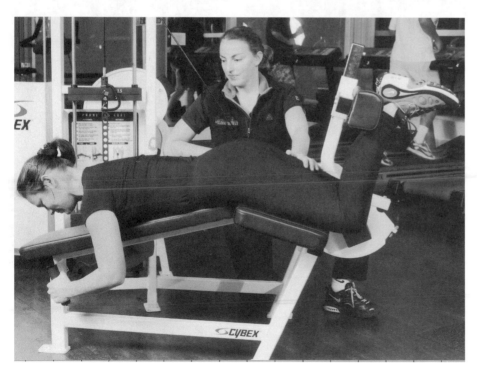

○ Overhead Shoulder Press

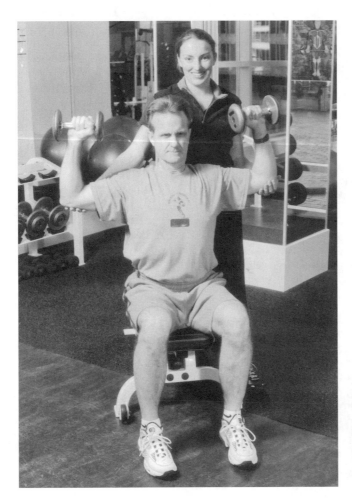

UPPER BODY

WORKS THE ANTERIOR AND MEDIAL DELTOIDS, TRICEPS

Sitting on a bench, grab a set of hand–weights and lift them up beside your shoulders so that your upper arms are parallel to the floor and your forearms are perpendicular to the floor. Press the weights upward until your elbows are fully extended but not locked. Slowly return to the starting position. Remember to keep your abdominals contracted and your torso stable throughout the exercise. Avoid allowing your shoulders to hunch upward. Perform a set of 8 to 12 or 10 to 15 reps. This is a compound movement.

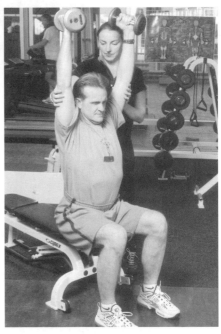

○ Calf Press

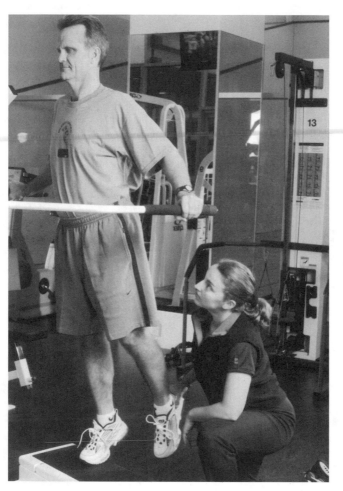

LOWER BODY

WORKS THE CALVES

Standing on one foot on a bench or step. Place your toes on the edge of the step so that your heels hang off the back. Push through your toes and raise your heels. Go as far as you can, so that you are pressing right through your big toes. Now slowly lower your heels past the step to an easy, comfortable, stretched position. Perform a set of 8 to 12 or 10 to 15 reps.

○ Bicep Curl on One Leg

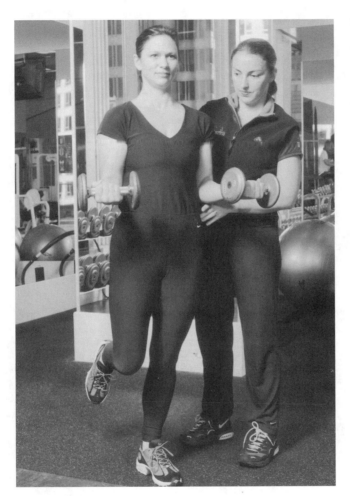

UPPER BODY

WORKS THE BICEPS, FOREARMS AND
ABDUCTORS

Grab a set of hand–weights. Keep
your chest out, shoulders back and
torso stable. Stand on one leg to
involve balance. Keeping the upper
arms stationary and your elbows at
your waist, bend at the elbow,
pulling the weights up toward your
shoulders. Try to avoid having your
elbows move forwards or backwards
— they should remain locked at
your side. Perform a set of 8 to 12
or 10 to 15 reps.

○ Tibialis Toe Pull

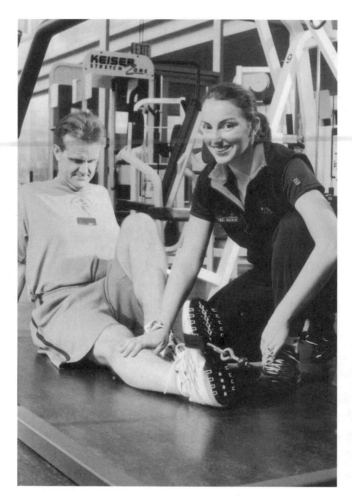

LOWER BODY

WORKS THE SHINS

Sit in front of a pulley system, with one leg bent and the other straight. Loop a strap around the top part of the foot of your straight leg. Be sure you are seated back far enough that you can feel the resistance on your shin muscle. Keeping your leg straight, pull your toes toward you as far as you can. Slowly release to the starting position. Perform a set of 8 to 12 or 10 to 15 reps for each leg.

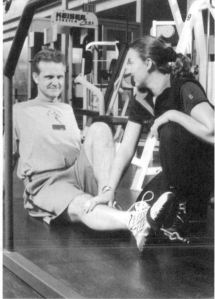

⊙ Tricep Press–down

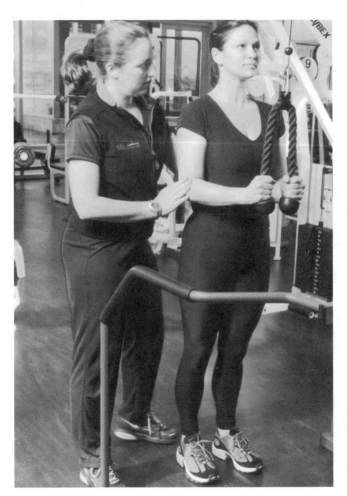

UPPER BODY

WORKS THE TRICEPS

Stand facing a pulley system, with a rope or bar attached to the top pulley. Grip the bar with your hands shoulder width apart, palms facing away, keeping your elbows locked by your side. Keep your abdominals contracted, chest up and out, shoulders down and back and torso stable. Keeping your elbows locked at your side, slowly push the bar downward until your arm is fully extended. Slowly release back to a 90–degree angle at the elbow. Perform a set of 8 to 12 or 10 to 15 reps.

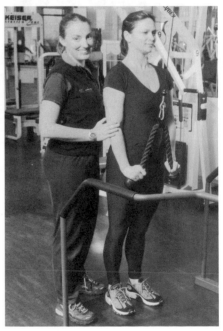

○ Inner Thigh Squeeze

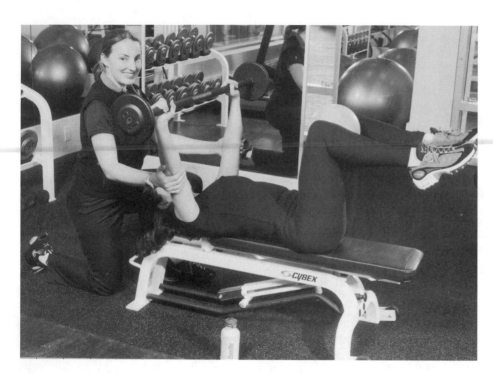

LOWER BODY

WORKS THE ADDUCTORS

The most common exercises for training the inner thigh muscles use a cable pulley with a kicking–across–the–body action, or those humiliating adductor/abductor machines that look all too similar to a gynecologist's stirrup contraption. But the adductor muscles actually function in our day–to–day lives as stabilizers and repositioners, not as movers! If we wanted to train those muscles more functionally, we'd train them in the same fashion that we use them.

The best way to do this is to train them while doing another movement. For example, while squatting, hold a medicine ball between your lower thighs/knees. This will force your adductors to contract isometrically to hold the ball in place. Or, while performing abdominal exercises, place a ball or a towel between your legs and keep your inner thighs contracted to hold it in place. Or, while performing any exercise while lying on your back, instead of having your legs relaxed suspend them in the air and hold a ball between your thighs. Training your inner thighs while you're performing other exercises mirrors how your body works in real life.

⊙ One–Legged Stance

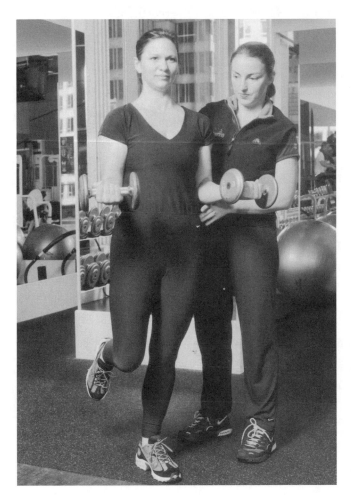

LOWER BODY

WORKS THE ABDUCTORS

When training the outer thigh muscles, most people resort to the cable pulley, the side–lying leg lifts or the stirrups. But in real life the abductors function as stabilizers and repositioners. The best way to challenge your outer thigh region functionally is the one–legged stance. When you stand on one leg, the tendency is to lean into that hip and hang off your hip ligaments. To level off your pelvis and regain neutral alignment, the gluteus medius muscle (your primary abductor) contracts to bring you into that position. Try standing on one leg for a minute or so with perfect posture and alignment. You'll notice that your outer thigh region will start to fatigue pretty quickly. I use this one–legged stance with my clients in any exercise they would normally do standing on two legs.

It works very well for lateral and anterior shoulder raises, bicep curls, tricep press–downs and overhead shoulder presses. This way you don't have to allocate an additional set of exercises for the outer thigh region.

COMBINATION EXERCISES

I want to give you some exercise ideas for incorporating combination training into your program. Try to include two or three of these types of exercises into each of your muscle strength and endurance workouts. I've increased the repetition zone to 13 to 20 reps for these exercises to allow you to focus more on muscle endurance.

○ Squat & Overhead Shoulder Press

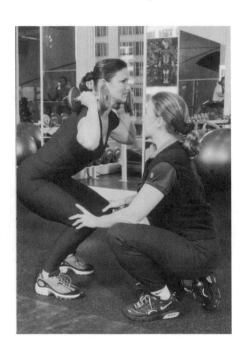 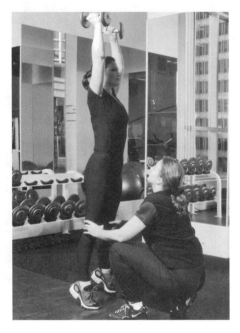

Stand with your feet between hip and shoulder width apart. Hold a set of hand-weights at shoulder height. Set your posture by contracting your abdominals, pressing your chest out and up and your shoulders back and down. Slowly squat backwards while keeping your kneecaps pointing forward. Lower until your upper thighs are parallel to the floor, or to a comfortable position. You'll notice that your upper body will come forward slightly. Now slowly extend upward while simultaneously lifting your hand-weights over your head. Perform one set of 13 to 20 reps.

⊙ Lunge and Lift & Lateral Shoulder Raise

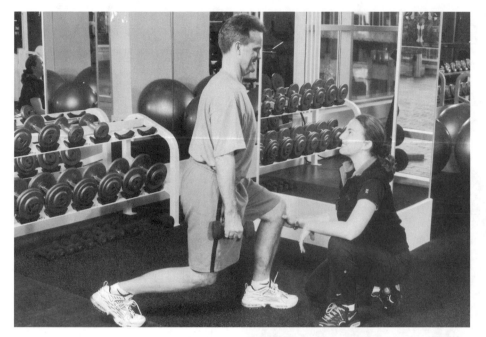

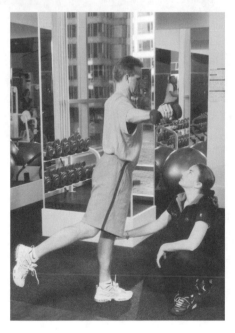

Start with one leg positioned in front of the other in a stride position while holding hand–weights at your sides. Keep your abdominals contracted and maintain good posture. Your front knee should remain above your front foot throughout the exercise, and this front leg should take the majority of your body weight and be your working leg. Lower slowly into a lunge position until your front upper thigh is parallel to the floor or until you hit a comfortable position. Now slowly extend upward, pushing off the front leg, until you are fully upright and balanced on the front leg. While pushing upward, lift your hand–weights to the side until they are at shoulder height. Then slowly lower back into the lunge position and release your arms to the side. Perform a set of 6 to 10 reps on each leg.

○ Step–Ups & Bicep Curls

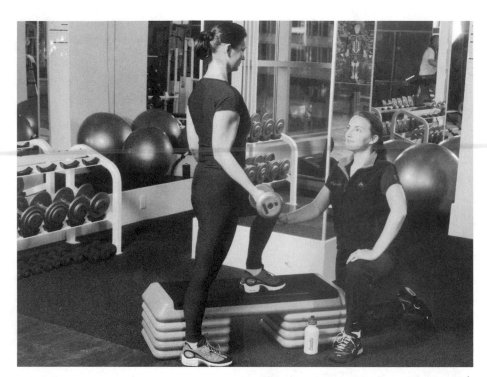

Position yourself in front of a crate or a staircase, with one foot on the second step. Holding hand–weights, keep your kneecap facing forward and your weight distributed on all four corners of your foot. Slowly step up, extending the supporting knee into a fully upright, balanced position. While extending upward, simultaneously curl your hand–weights toward your shoulders, keeping your elbows at your sides. Then slowly lower yourself to the starting position. Perform a set of 6 to 10 reps on each leg.

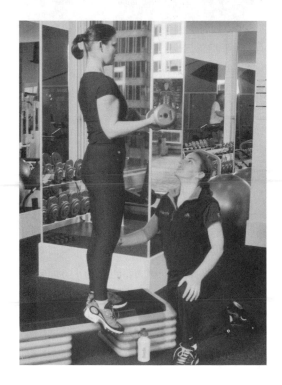

○ Chest Press & Leg Lifts

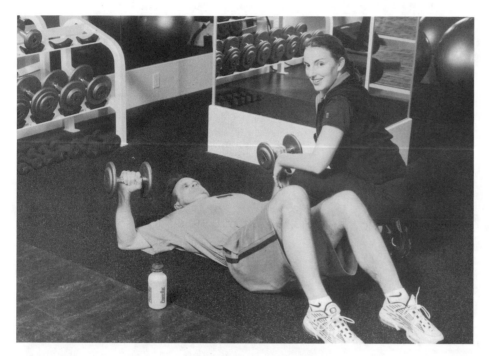

Holding free weights, lie on your back with your knees bent and feet flat on the floor. Bend your legs more for an easier version or keep them straight for a more difficult option. Start with your elbows bent at your sides at shoulder height and your hands positioned over your elbows. Slowly press the hand–weights upward until your elbows are fully extended. At the same time, slowly lift onc leg a few inches off the floor while keeping your abdominals contracted and your back in a stable and neutral position. Perform a set of 13 to 20 reps.

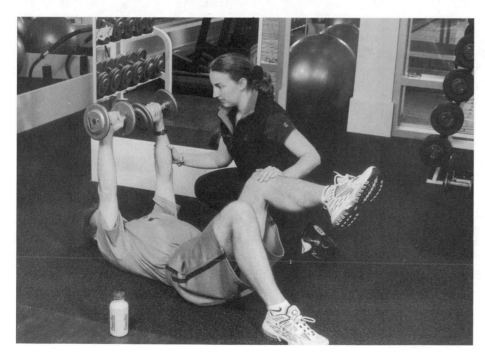

○ Leg Lowers & Tricep Extension

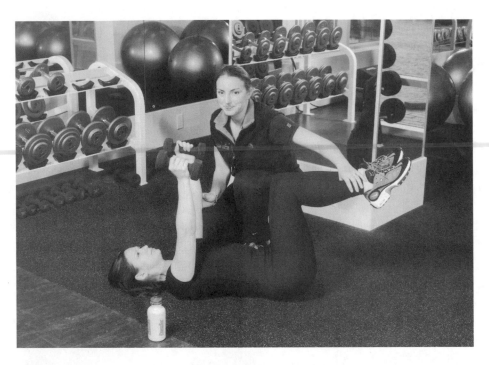

Lie on your back with your feet suspended in the air, so that your upper thighs are perpendicular to the floor and your lower legs are parallel to the floor (90–degree angle at your hips and knees). Keep your knees a few inches apart. Keep your abdominals pulled inward throughout the exercise, and your back neutral and completely stable. Hold hand–weights and position your arms so that they are extended toward the ceiling and your wrists and elbows are positioned over your shoulders. Now slowly bend your elbows so that your hand–weights lower toward the top of your head. As you lower the hand–weights, lower one leg toward the floor. While that leg is moving, the other is completely stable. Your back should not move throughout the exercise. Perform a set of 13 to 20 reps.

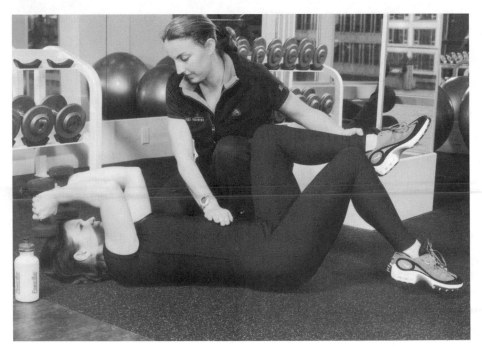

Aerobic & Anaerobic Cardiovascular Exercise with Variable Impact & Agility Training

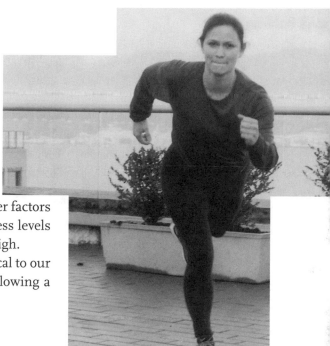

Dr. Steven Blair and his colleagues at the Cooper Fitness Institute in Dallas, Texas, did the largest study to date focusing on fitness. They recruited more than 25,000 men and more than 7,000 women aged 20 to 88. Subjects were followed for seven to eight years and underwent extensive physical exams, including treadmill testing. Height, weight, blood pressure, cholesterol levels, smoking habits and medical histories were collected. The biggest difference between the 601 men and 89 women who died during the follow-up period and those who didn't was not fatness but fitness. When other factors were taken into account, it was found that those with the lowest fitness levels had double the mortality rate of those whose fitness was medium or high.

Dr. Blair's study indicates clearly that cardiovascular fitness is critical to our overall health and fitness. Some specific benefits associated with following a regular cardiovascular conditioning program are:

- Aerobic capacity increased by 30 per cent.

- Increased bone density. In one controlled study of 25 women aged 49 to 61, lumbar spine bone mineral density was significantly higher in those who jogged or played volleyball than in those who had no regular physical activity. A 12-month study of more than 200 postmenopausal women found that those who walked 12 kilometers (7.5 miles) per week had a higher average bone mineral density of the trunk, legs and whole body than those who walked less than 1.6 kilometers (one mile) per week.

- Improved body composition. A cross-sectional study of female athletes and sedentary women aged 18 to 69 found no difference in body fat percentage and fat-free mass between the youngest and older athletes; in addition, the resting metabolic rate of the older exercisers was closer to that of the young athletes than to that of sedentary, age-matched women. Another study followed 507 women, aged 42 to 50, for three years. Those who were least active at baseline and those whose activity declined during the study period gained the most weight.

- Reduced risk for coronary artery disease. Population studies have generally shown a strong inverse relationship between physical activity and heart disease risk and between cardiorespiratory fitness and risk of heart disease. While much of this research has focused on men, the findings are generally the same for women. For example, a study of nearly 1,500 Swedish women aged 38 to 60 found that those who were inactive during leisure time were nearly three times as likely to have coronary artery disease as those who were active; an eight year study of more than 3,000 women showed that an increase in aerobic capacity resulted in a decrease in the risk of death from cardiovascular disease.

- A natural high, and improved energy, enhanced sleep quality, improved posture, improved functional ability, improved sexual patterns, reduced episodes of depression.

- Reduced hot flashes and night sweats. A controlled, cross–sectional, population–based study of more than 1,600 women found that sedentary women were twice as likely to report hot flashes as physically active women.

I'm including aerobic and anaerobic cardiovascular exercise with variable impact as the strategy for slowing the aging process. Let's examine each of these components.

Aerobic exercise is easy to explain. It involves going out for a walk, jog, cycle or swim or taking a fitness class. It's exercise that is within your comfort zone and performed at an intensity that you can hold for 20 or more minutes. This type of exercise conditions your heart and achieves the benefits listed above.

Anaerobic exercise is a more challenging form of exercise. It involves the same activities as aerobic exercise but at a much harder intensity. For example, it might mean going for a jog, then picking up the pace and sprinting, for 30 seconds, then returning to the easier intensity. You could do this at regular intervals during a running, cycling, swimming or walking workout. This kind of workout really helps you get fit fast. It raises what is called your anaerobic or respiratory threshold. This threshold point is the feeling you experience during an activity session when you're pushing hard. You start to breathe really heavily, and your heart pounds fast. If you hold this pace for too long, you might start to feel nauseated and dizzy. This is one of the side effects of lactic acid buildup — a by–product of high–intensity exercise.
When you perform anaerobic intervals as described above, you hold the more intense pace only for 30 seconds to two minutes, and just before you're about

to start experiencing some of those nasty side effects of high–intensity exercise, you drop the pace and allow your body to recover. By doing these brief, high–intensity intervals, your body becomes accustomed to them and is better able to handle the lactic acid, flush it out of the tissues and actually use it for energy. By doing anaerobic intervals you will get fit fast, and you'll start to notice that intensities that used to get you huffing and puffing aren't that challenging any more. This form of interval conditioning will also expend more calories per minute and help you achieve your fat–loss goals.

A NOTE: If you are a beginner, wait a few months and exercise at a moderate rate before graduating to high–intensity exercise. Of course, the faster you walk, step, dance, cycle or run, the more calories you use per minute. However, if you have been sedentary high–intensity exercise compromises your ability to sustain exercise for a long time. For that reason, lower–intensity exercise is more effective in the initial stages of training and is a prerequisite for higher–calorie–burning, higher–intensity exercise. In fact, you will experience great results by just getting started on a program. You do not want to start by dreading each exercise session because you know it is going to hurt; that will make it difficult to stay motivated. Three easy walks a week on an ongoing basis is far better than one hard run every once in a while.

Remember, consistency is the key to getting results. You are going to want to eventually intensify your program and make a good effort at each workout, but progress to this level slowly. Start with two months of easy training with a slow, gradual progression. Do not worry about intensity. Just work on increasing the amount of time you spend exercising. You may, for example, initially structure only two cardio sessions per week for one to two months. Progress from there, incorporating another session each week until you reach the American College of Sports Medicine recommendations of three to five cardio workouts each week.

"Variable impact" refers to exposing your body to a bit of impact here and there. It is important because in order to maintain muscle mass and bone density you need to apply a little bit of stress to the bone. You may have heard many people complain that high–impact exercise really bothers their joints, specifically their back, knees or feet. For a lot of people, high–impact activity may not be the exercise of choice. However, in your program you want to ensure that you do expose your muscles and bones to some impact. So, for example, if your main exercise is swimming, since your body weight is supported by the water you should complement swimming with an activity such as walking. Swimming is a great activity, but recent studies have shown that it

> "Old age is not a time of life. It is a condition of the body. It is not time that ages the body, it is abuse that does…"
>
> — HERBERT M. SHELTON

is not as beneficial for bone density as medium–impact (e.g., walking) or high–impact activities (e.g., volleyball). Though swimming is better than no exercise, it should be augmented with strength training or a type of activity that will provide a bit more impact. If you'd like to try jogging, stick to a walk/run program in which you start, for example, with walking for four minutes and running for only one minute at a time. This will be sufficient to provide positive results.

Finally, try to incorporate *agility training* into your workouts. We know that as we get older our fast–twitch muscle fibers atrophy, which is one reason why someone who is older moves more slowly. To slow this rate of decline, a program that includes agility training is important. This keeps you mobile and agile as you age. I will include some agility exercise ideas at the end of this subsection.

Cardiovascular Prescription

A U.S. surgeon general's report in 1996 suggested that 30 minutes of light activity every day (equivalent to doing household chores, walking, gardening, cycling) will be sufficient to improve someone's health. This is a nonstructured way of attempting to improve your health. All you have to do is commit to being more active in your life. Just try to get in 30 minutes of activity every day.

If your goals are a bit more aggressive and you really desire to improve your overall fitness, your prescription will require a higher level of volume and intensity.

The American College of Sports Medicine recommends 20 to 60 minutes of cardiovascular activity three to five days a week to maximize fitness.

The type of aerobic activity must be continuous and involve your large muscle groups. Some of the best choices are:

- Walking
- Running
- Cycling
- Swimming
- In–line skating
- Hiking
- Rowing
- Racquet sports
- Cross–country skiing
- Stair climbing
- Fitness classes

> "A healthy body is a guest-chamber for the soul; a sick body is a prison."
>
> — FRANCIS BACON

Choosing an Aerobic Activity

The most important consideration when choosing your primary activity is whether you like it and so will stick with it. The best activity in the world is the one you do regularly. If I told you that running was the best way to get in shape but you hated running, you probably would not stick to a running program very well and would have limited results. So you really need to examine your interests. If you prefer to exercise outside, running along trails or hiking may be your answer. If you prefer to be indoors, you might enjoy the energy of fitness classes, or working out on a stair climber while you read a magazine or watch TV. If you like to exercise in groups, fitness classes or a walking clinic may help you stick to your program. It is important to determine the perfect–fit, custom–designed program that will facilitate your efforts.

When deciding whether an activity is the right one for you, ask yourself the following questions:

- Do I like it? Is it fun?
- Is it interesting? Is it stimulating?
- Do I get absorbed in it?
- Do I feel energized during and/or after it? Invigorated? Refreshed?
- Does it give me a sense of accomplishment?

If you answered "yes" to all these questions, you've made a good choice. If you've answered "no" to most and you find the activity unpleasant, boring or frustrating and hate every second of it, you should search for an alternative that will provide you with more enjoyment.

Remember that consistency is the key to achieving your exercise goals. Find an activity you enjoy and you will be motivated to participate more consistently and reap the benefits more quickly. Find the activity that sparks your interest and soon you will enjoy a fit and healthier body.

Designing Your Weekly Cardiovascular Program

Structure two to three long but easy–intensity workouts each week. These sessions should be at least 45 minutes in duration and involve a rating of perceived exertion (RPE) intensity of 5. (You'll learn about RPE monitoring at the end of this subsection.) These workouts will definitely feel very comfortable. You may even feel that you are going too slowly. You are not! Workouts in this zone are not very stressful on your body but will effectively challenge and overload your aerobic energy system and help to develop fat–burning enzymes. This intensity zone is recommended if you are just getting started to exercise.

The other zones may be too stressful and uncomfortable for you at this point.

Structure one to two moderate–length and medium–intensity aerobic workouts each week. These sessions should last for 30 or 40 minutes and involve an RPE effort level of 6 to 7. This is the intensity zone where most people will train, so it will feel comfortable. Most people neglect training in the extreme zones — the very easy and the very challenging.

Structure one to two short and intense interval workouts each week. These workouts should last for approximately 20 minutes and should involve an RPE intensity of approximately 8. During these workouts you will notice that your breathing is heavier and your heart is beating more quickly. These sessions will definitely be above the comfort zone in which you would prefer to exercise.

Include a six to 12 minute low–intensity warm–up and cooldown. The body does not respond very well to going from inactivity to very intense activity. The cardiovascular, musculoskeletal, neurological and metabolic energy pathways need to be stimulated gradually in order to perform at an optimal level. Muscles that are warm have a much better ability to extract and utilize oxygen to produce energy. As muscles warm up, the enzyme activity level is increased. This means that fats and sugars are broken down more rapidly, and more energy and less lactic acid (the burning sensation) will be produced. This will enhance your performance and increase your ability to burn fat. Exercisers in their later years may need an even more extensive warm–up of approximately 15 minutes.

Your body also does not respond very well to going from intense activity to complete rest. Your heart, lungs, muscles, joints and energy systems require a gradual cool–down to avoid dizziness or blood pooling in the lower extremities, and to assist in the recovery process. In addition, warming up and cooling down is a way to prolong your caloric burn for each workout. So, for example, if you are going to go for a run, start with a six–minute walk. Then start a light jog and work into your normal running pace. When you've completed your workout, finish with a six–minute cooling walk and then stretch. A warm–up and cooldown should generally involve the same workout activity but at a much lower intensity.

"Enjoy the seasons of life ... Each season of life is wonderful if you have learned the lessons of the season before. It is only when you go on with lessons unlearned that you wish for a return..."

— PEACE PILGRIM

Working out indoors? Use a variety of machines. If you are using indoor car-diovascular machines, stay on the same one for a maximum of 10 to 15 min-utes. Using a variety of machines will create better muscle balance. I would rather see someone spend 10 minutes each on the step machine, rowing machine, treadmill and ski machine than spend 40 minutes just on the step machine. If you are using the same machine or activity all the time, the mus-cles targeted will continue to get fitter but other, neglected muscles will not. Muscle imbalances are sure to surface. Varying your training will develop a more toned physique overall and reduce your risk of injury.

Varying your indoor machines also will help to prevent boredom. I have no difficulty going for a two–hour bike ride outside, but get me on a stationary bike and after 10 minutes I am stir–crazy! If you're working out at home and have only one indoor machine, perhaps mix up your program. For example, you could start by walking on the treadmill for 15 minutes, then get off the machine for a few minutes and skip or step up and down onto a step, then get back onto the treadmill to finish your workout.

Structure at least one recovery day into your weekly exercise program. Remember this: muscle tissue does not grow stronger during exercise. In fact, muscle breaks down during exercise! It needs a period of recovery to repair, grow, develop and get stronger. Back–to–back hard workouts mean the muscles never get a chance to fully recover. Incorporating one to two recovery days into your workout week will ensure your body gets a chance to heal. Do not think, though, that you need to stay home, chained to your couch and TV. When I say "recovery," I mean that maybe you go for an easy stroll or hike or cycle, but you are not concerned about getting into your training zone. These are the days you just enjoy life and take time to experience simpler pursuits.

Remember also to consider your lifestyle. How many days per week do you think you can commit to exercise? What time of the day works best for you? Which days will work best to exercise and which to take as rest days?

Measuring Intensity

Many exercisers ask whether they are working too hard or should be breaking more of a sweat. How do you know if you are exercising in the right intensity zones? This is where monitoring your heart rate comes in. Traditionally, an intensity of 70 per cent of your maximum heart rate was thought to be the ideal. But this one–size–fits–all approach might not provide the best results for everyone. A more custom–designed approach is more effective. Here is how to go about it.

First, determine which of the following zones fits your goals: general health, weight management, aerobic conditioning, advanced conditioning or a combination of all four.

Zone 1: General health. A great deal of research indicates that being active at 50 to 60 per cent of your maximum heart rate, consistently and for a total of 30 minutes on most days, reduces the risk of developing many chronic diseases. Low–intensity activities such as walking, gardening, household chores or easy cycling will achieve this. If someone does not need to lose body fat and is not training for a sporting event, this may be all he or she needs to do to stay healthy.

Zone 2: Weight management. If your goal is to reduce body fat and you have been relatively inactive, you will need to train at a level of 60 to 70 per cent of your maximum heart rate. This is still within your comfort zone and allows you to exercise at a steady pace for long enough to burn off a substantial number of calories.

Zone 3: Aerobic conditioning/weight management. If your goal is to improve your cardiovascular conditioning for better stamina and endurance, you should train within a zone of 70 to 80 per cent of your maximum heart rate. This is also a good zone for fat burning if you are already fairly fit. This zone requires a more vigorous level of activity.

Zone 4: Advanced conditioning. If you are in top shape and training for a sporting event such as a 10–kilometer race, a triathlon or tennis match, you might need to include some workouts at 80 per cent of your maximum heart rate or higher. This level of training is both physically and mentally demanding, so it is not something you would do on a daily basis. And it is not for everyone. Only the advanced exerciser should consider working in this range. This zone is also a fat–burning zone if you are extremely fit.

Ideally, your exercise program will include workouts in each of these ranges — short and hard to long and easy. So how do you determine whether you're in the right zone during any given workout? Here is a formula to help you figure it out.

First you must determine your true resting heart rate. Before you get up in the morning, measure your heart rate for one minute. Be sure to wait a few minutes after the alarm has gone off, so that your heart will recover from being startled. Do this for three days in a row and take the average of all three. This is your resting heart rate.

"A man is not old until regrets take the place of dreams…"

— John Barrymore

Homework

1. **Determine your true resting heart rate (RHR).**

   Day 1:   _____ beats per minute

   Day 2:   _____ beats per minute

   Day 3:   _____ beats per minute

   Average resting heart rate =   _____ beats per minute

2. **Determine your estimated maximum heart rate (MHR).**

   Females   = 226 minus age = _____

   Males   = 220 minus age = _____

   The age–adjusted MHR formula is perfect for our purposes, although a more accurate method is to determine your MHR in a laboratory setting using a stress test administrated by a physician or sports physiologist. These tests are generally done on a treadmill or exercise bicycle and cost between $100 and $300. Assuming you don't want to spend the money on a maximal heart rate test, the formula above will work just fine.

3. **Determine which of the four previously discussed training zones you'd like to calculate (general health, weight management, aerobic conditioning/weight management, advanced conditioning).**

4. **Determine the low end of your training zone.**

   Low end of training zone =
   [(MHR minus RHR) × _____%] + RHR = _____ beats per minute (bpm)

5. **Determine the high end of your training zone.**

   High end of training zone =
   [(MHR minus RHR) × _____%] + RHR = _____ beats per minute

   Your optimal training zone is _____ beats per minute.

Let's take as an example a 40–year–old inactive woman who wants to lose body fat. Let's say we've determined that her resting heart rate in the morning is 70 beats per minute (bpm).

⊙ Her estimated maximum heart rate = 226 bpm minus age (40) = 186 bpm.

⊙ Low end of training zone = [(MHR {186 bpm} minus RHR {70 bpm} × 60%] + 70 bpm = 140 beats per minute.

⊙ High end of training zone = [(MHR {186 bpm} minus RHR {70 bpm} × 70%] + 70 bpm = 151 beats per minute.

We see she needs to train at a heart rate of 140 to 151 beats per minute.

Once you have determined your optimal training zones for each workout, the best way to ensure that you are in the correct zone is to invest in and use a heart rate monitor. This will provide an accurate, quick analysis of your heart rate and let you easily intensify or reduce the intensity of your workout if you are not in the right zone. Unfortunately, manual heart rate monitoring (counting your heart rate by placing your fingers on an artery in your wrist or neck) has been found to be inaccurate, with errors as high as 27 beats per minute. In addition, when testing on your neck or wrist you have to interrupt your workout to do the reading. I strongly encourage you to acquire a heart rate monitor. It will improve the effectiveness of your cardio workouts.

Although I regularly use battery–operated heart rate monitors with my clients, they have their drawbacks. Your heart rate can be affected by variables such as food, medication, temperature and stress, so it is necessary to monitor the intensity of your workouts with an additional indicator, the rating of perceived exertion (RPE) scale.

A New Scale to Measure Intensity

Rating of perceived exertion (RPE) is a scale that calls on your own perception of the intensity of a workout to indicate whether you are training in the appropriate zone. RPE is gaining popularity because of its effectiveness, simplicity and safety. The RPE scale was developed by Dr. Gunnar Borg of Sweden. Dr. Borg noticed a close relationship between an athlete's exercising heart rate (which is directly related to the intensity of the exercise) and how the athlete perceived his or her effort. The original Borg method used a scale from 6 to

20. It has since been modified to a more user–friendly scale from 0 to 10. Zero on the scale represents a resting level with no elevation in breathing. At the other extreme, a rating of 10 indicates all–out effort and severe exhaustion. Here is how to match up the numbers with your workouts.

0 Represents a resting level, with no elevation in your breathing.

1 Represents a more active rest, such as working at your desk, with no elevation in your breathing.

2 Represents an active resting level, such as getting dressed or walking around in your house, with no elevation in your breathing.

3 Represents a low level of activity, such as gardening or the warm–up stages in a workout. You may be aware of your breathing, but it is slow and natural.

4 Represents a low level of activity, such as a stroll or an easy bike ride, with a slight elevation in breathing. You are still well within your comfort zone. This is your predominant training zone for your warm–up or your entire workout if you fall within the general health training zone (50 to 60 per cent MHR).

5 Represents a moderate level of activity, such as walking briskly. Your breathing is elevated higher than in level 4, but you are still well within your comfort zone. This is your predominant training zone if you fall within the weight management training zone, or if you were scheduled for a long, easy workout (60 to 70 per cent MHR).

6 Represents a moderate level of activity, such as walking briskly to an appointment for which you are very late. Your breathing is faster and deeper, but you are within your comfort zone. You feel that you can comfortably hold a conversation. This is still within your weight management training zone or your moderate–intensity workout zone (60 to 70 per cent MHR).

7 Represents a more vigorous level of activity, such as jogging. Your breathing is more rapid and deep, and you feel you could hold a conversation but would prefer not to. This intensity is beginning to feel more challenging and outside your comfort zone. This is your predominant training zone if you fall within the aerobic conditioning/weight management zone or are performing a moderate–intensity workout (70 to 80 per cent MHR).

"The purpose of life… is to live, to taste experience to the utmost, to reach out eagerly and without fear for newer and richer experience."

— ELEANOR ROOSEVELT

8 Represents a vigorous level of activity, such as faster running. You could hold a conversation, but it would be short. You think you can continue for the remainder of your session, but you are not 100 per cent confident that you can make it. You feel that you are outside your comfort zone and being heavily challenged. This is still your aerobic conditioning/weight management training zone (70 to 80 per cent MHR).

9 Represents a very, very vigorous level of activity, such as incorporating sprinting intervals in a run. Your breathing is very labored and you could not hold a conversation. You would definitely feel fatigued and outside of your comfort zone. This is your predominant training zone if you fall within the advanced conditioning zone or are performing a short, hard workout (80 per cent or more MHR).

10 Represents an all–out effort, with severe exhaustion. It is not recommended that you train at this level.

During your workouts, check regularly to ensure that, on the scale of 0 to 10, you're exercising at the right level. For example, let's say you are a regular exerciser and you'd like to perform a 40–minute moderate–level workout with the goal of maximizing fat loss. Start with a six to 12–minute warm–up at an RPE level of 3 or 4. Then pick up the pace for 40 minutes and maintain an RPE level of 6 or 7. During the workout your breathing is relatively fast and deep, but you are still within your comfort zone. You feel that you could comfortably hold a conversation during the entire 40 minutes but you prefer not to do so. When you're done, finish off with a cooldown at an intensity of 3 or 4.

Agility Training Ideas
Here are some ideas to help you maintain agility and mobility as you age. Try to perform one agility drill once or twice each week.

◎ Lateral Agility Drill

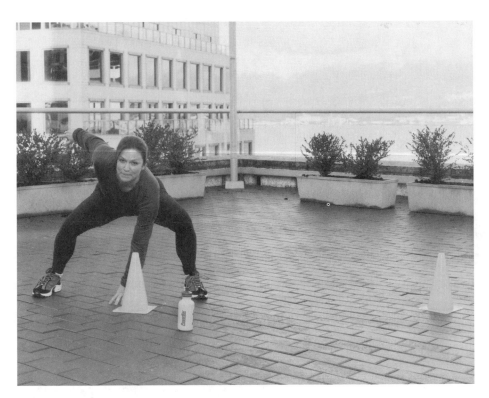

Position two cones or props such as chairs or books a few feet apart. Quickly step laterally to the outside of one cone and back to the outside of the other, touching down toward the floor at each end. Try to go as fast as you can. Continue for 30 seconds.

○ Sprint Drills

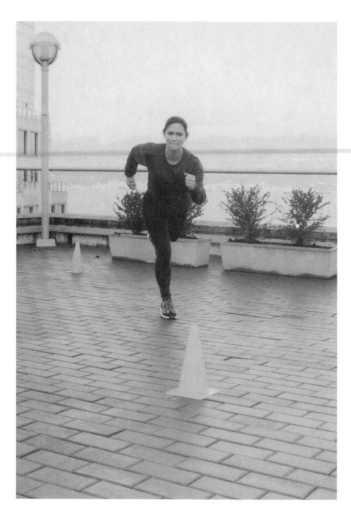

Place three cones in a straight line, about 50 feet apart. You can also use telephone poles on a road or driveways on your street. Start the exercise by sprinting or walking fast to the first cone, then shuffle backwards to the starting point. Sprint to the second cone, then shuffle backwards to the starting point. Sprint all the way to the third cone, then shuffle backwards to the starting point. Take a short break and then repeat this 5 or 10 times.

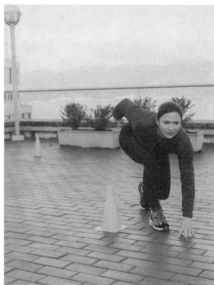

◎ Rectangle Drill

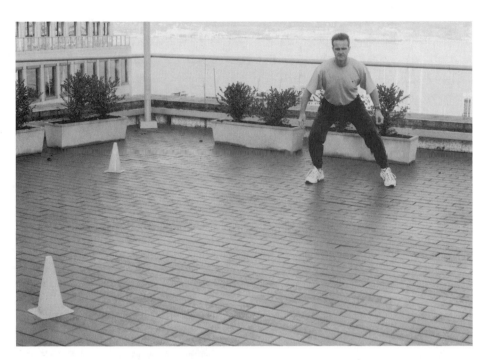

Place four cones in the shape of a rectangle or square, with each cone about 30 feet from the next. Start at one corner and sprint to the top of the square. Shuffle across the top of the square. Back–shuffle. Laterally shuffle back to the start. Do this 5 times in one direction. Take a break and go in the reverse direction. You can also use the lines on a tennis court to perform this drill.

An easy way to incorporate agility training into your exercise program is by participating in activities such as squash, tennis, racquetball, basketball and volleyball, or by enrolling in dance programs such as salsa or ballroom dancing, or in choreography–based fitness classes such as funk and hip–hop. These types of activities will keep you agile and mobile into your later years — and they're fun.

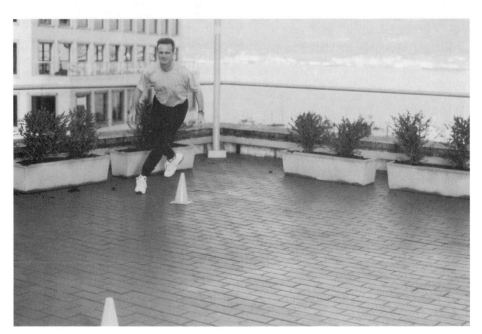

It's important that you realize you do not need to implement all of my suggestions today. You might choose to start by just committing to exercising three times per week. Once you have made that a habit, you can mix up the intensity zones by incorporating one easy, one moderate and one hard workout into each week. A few months later, you can incorporate a different type of activity. A few months after that, you can invest in a heart rate monitor and start seriously monitoring your zones.

The beautiful part of this program is that you have designed it. You are your own personal trainer and at any time you can modify, restructure or adjust, depending on your rate of success, enjoyment and adherence.

Postural, Abdominal & Back Training

I bet you're thinking that we covered muscle conditioning in the previous strategy, and you're right, we did. But we neglected to discuss some essential areas. The exercises in this subsection are very important and specific to helping reverse some of the changes most people experience as they get older. Many complain of knee, shoulder and back pain. We will now take a proactive approach to helping you minimize the chances of having to endure debilitating deterioration in these areas.

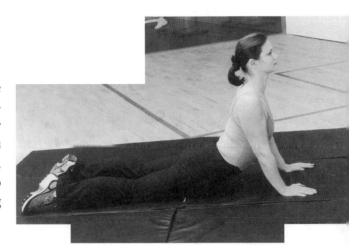

Postural Training

"Stand up straight!" "Don't slouch!" Your momma was right. Posture is important because it helps your body function at top performance in all situations. If you have ever felt instant agony the moment you bent over to pick up something, you can't blame the load for the pain you're experiencing. Most back problems originate from years of abuse through slouching in front of the TV, hunching over a desk, lifting and bending improperly, using poor posture and maintaining a sedentary lifestyle. Consider the fellow who suffers a heart attack while shoveling snow: He has experienced years and years of bad eating habits, stress and a sedentary lifestyle and those are to blame for the heart attack, not the snow. In the same way, a lifetime of poor posture and poor lifting and bending habits might stress the spine to the point that, one day, a minor thing like sneezing, slight twisting or bending over might precipitate extreme back pain.

If you have poor posture, your bones are not properly aligned and your muscles, joints and ligaments take more strain than intended. Try this experiment: Bend your thumb backwards as far as you can and hold it there for as long as you can. Eventually you're going to feel some pain. But an X-ray wouldn't show any trauma and a biopsy wouldn't reveal an infection. The pain comes from holding the thumb in an extreme, uncomfortable position. Once the thumb returns to its normal position, the pain goes away.

Back pain is similar. Years of poor posture place the back in an extreme, uncomfortable position that causes muscle fatigue, muscular strain and eventually pain. By returning the back to its neutral position of comfort through exercise and posture retraining, the pain should slowly subside. If this isn't enough to persuade you to correct your posture, remember this — good posture contributes to a better appearance and a sense of confidence and poise.

Standing Posture

So how do you get good posture? Well, first you need to be aware when you're not in proper postural alignment. I want you to imagine that you have a piece of thread that runs through your body from head to toe, linking the bones and muscles in proper alignment. Whenever your posture is poor, you can simply pull gently on the top of the thread and it will realign your body perfectly.

Here's what good posture looks like when the thread is tight:

- The head is centered over the trunk, with the chin level and held over the collarbone. The gaze is level. The ears are in line with the tips of the shoulders.

- The shoulders are aligned over the hips and are held slightly back, down and relaxed. The shoulder blades are flat.

- The arms hang loosely, with the palms facing the sides of the body.

- The chest is up and open; the rib cage feels as if it is expanded and well anchored against the spine.

- The back feels long and strong, slightly curved in the lower region.

- The abdomen is pulled in and up.

- The pelvis is tilted slightly up so that the buttocks feel tucked under but relaxed. Imagine your pelvis to be a full bowl of water: if you tip it forward too far, the water will spill out the front, and if you tip it backwards too far, the water will spill out the back.

- The knees are straight and relaxed, neither bent nor hyperextended.

- The feet are parallel, slightly apart, with weight balanced evenly among the heels and the outside borders and balls of the feet.

Awareness of this posture is critical in helping you change any misalignments. One of the common postural deviations I deal with is the shoulders rounded forward and the upper back in a kyphotic (slight hunchback) position. When I put such a client into neutral postural alignment, it feels awkward and it should — she's been used to abnormal posture for often 40 or more years. It'll take some time for the right posture to feel right. Be persistent. Every time you pass a mirror, do a self–check. Or have a friend or loved one correct you when he or she notices you're slouching. The keys to improving your posture are awareness and a consistent effort to maintain proper alignment.

Sitting Posture

People who sit a lot in their jobs are at highest risk for low–back pain, because the highest measured pressure inside the disk occurs when sitting. If your job involves hours of sitting, set an alarm at your desk to remind you every half hour to stand up and walk around the office or do a few stretches. It'll take only a few seconds to get blood flowing back into your spinal region and relieve some of the strain to which extended sitting exposes your body.

Another option to ease extended sitting is to use a lumbar roll or cushion, available at any medical supply shop. This type of passive support will help keep the natural curve in your lower back and reduce your symptoms. But keep in mind that only active conditioning through exercise will develop the muscles you need for a truly healthy back.

If you find yourself in a seated posture for a long period, stand up, place your hands on your lower back and slowly bend backwards while looking toward the ceiling. Hold for five seconds. Repeat 5 times.

To find your correct sitting posture, first sit in a really slouched position, then slowly straighten your back and arch it. Immediately relax the arch in your lower back by about 10 per cent. This is your neutral back position and correct sitting posture. If your posture isn't ideal, you might find at first that your muscles will tire quickly from trying to maintain this position. That's okay. Eventually, as with any exercise, you'll get better at it.

To further alleviate some of the strain of having to sit for extended periods, at the end of a long day and just before bed try these stretches.

○ Back Extension

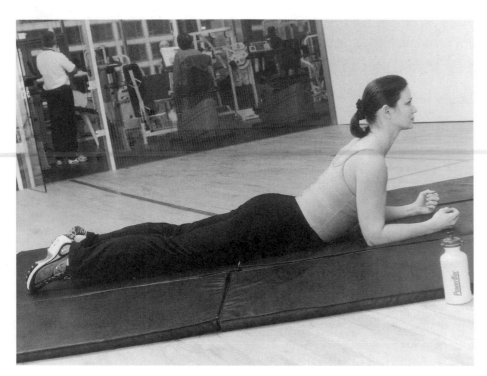

Lie on your stomach and prop your upper body onto your elbows. Keep your hips on the floor and relax your lower back. Try to imagine your ribs stretching away from your hips. Hold for about 30 seconds. Repeat 3 to 5 times.

○ Advanced Back Extension Stretch

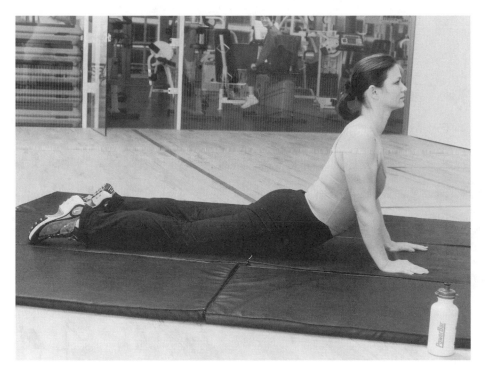

Lie on your stomach, with your palms near your shoulders as if preparing to perform a push–up. Slowly, using your upper body muscles, push your shoulders up, keeping your hips on the floor and letting your back arch. Hold for five seconds. Repeat 3 to 5 times.

○ Pillow Arch

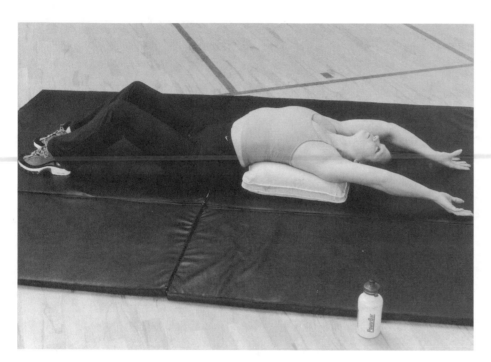

Place two to three pillows on the floor, one on top of the other. Lie on your back over the pillows, so that the pillows are at about the level of your shoulder blades. Stretch your arms over your head and just relax. Hold the stretch for at least one minute.

Abdominal Training

Abdominal crunches have become the gold standard of abdominal exercises, but they may not be doing as much as we think to give us the strong torso we need to play sports, walk, lift or perform other daily activities.

The problem is in the movement. In an abdominal crunch we perform, technically speaking, a forward flexion of the spine. But many of us spend the entire day in a forward–flexed position. We sit forward at desks, sit forward at a computer, sit flexed to watch TV, sit flexed to drive, sit flexed at a table to eat. Why would we want to strengthen our body in a direction that we really should be trying to avoid? Think of the typical posture of someone who is aging: They start to round more and more forward into that hunchback posture. It makes sense that we'd want to try to counteract and minimize these forward forces. I'm not suggesting that you shouldn't be doing any abdominal crunches, but if you choose to do any crunch exercises they should be a minimal aspect of your abdominal–conditioning program. Instead, you should focus on more functional and appropriate movements such as the ones at the end of this subsection.

The key to the health of your back is understanding the concept of co–contraction, that is, the muscles of the abdominal region must work together with the muscles along the back of your spine to keep your spine stabilized. The abdominal musculature in most people does not do its job. It is in a weak, relaxed state all day long, and so the load of stabilizing the spine is taken through our back musculature. It is no wonder that 80 per cent of us will suffer back pain at some point in our life. The good news is that 90 per cent of lower–back problems are preventable. All you have to do is make a focused effort to strengthen the muscles that will help minimize muscle imbalances and promote better posture.

Here's how you can start developing a healthy back today.

DAILY ABDOMINAL CONTRACTIONS

If you decide you'd like to condition your abs, you might do a couple of sets of crunches three times per week. This might take you five minutes each time for a total of 15 minutes of work each week. My question is this: what are you doing in the other 167 hours and 45 minutes of each week? A couple of sets of crunches a few times a week will do you no good if you're countering the benefits by using poor posture all day long.

One of the things I teach my clients right from the beginning is that if they want to condition their abdominals and minimize the chance of developing back pain they must start using their abs all day long. I start by asking them to contract their abdominals for 30 seconds. Most people will suck in their gut as hard as they can, and by the end of 30 seconds they're almost blue. Unfortunately, this isn't going to do them any good because, if they're contracting maximally, they're not going to be able to hold their abdominals in for very long. But we need them all day long. We need the kind of endurance that will allow us to sit all day behind a desk or stand for eight hours behind a counter or play with our kids or carry heavy groceries. So I ask my clients to contract their abdominals again, but this time only submaximally. The contraction should be at about 25 per cent of their maximal effort. The muscles are contracted just enough to pull the abdominal cavity inward. After about 30 seconds the muscles will generally get tired and the client will relax them. The abdominal cavity will pop out and protrude again.

I ask clients to do these types of abdominal contractions all day long — whenever they think about it. I ask them to use triggers. For example, every time the phone rings, suck in the abs. Every time they're stopped at a red light, suck in. When they're making dinner, suck in. I ask them to start with 30 seconds and then build up to one minute, then two minutes, and so on. Eventually the abdominal musculature will gain enough endurance to start doing its job — stabilizing the spine — all day long. The contraction of the abdominals will become part of normal posture. In fact, when the muscle is not pulling the abdominal cavity inward it will feel unnatural. This is what you want to achieve. Trust me, it works.

Abdominal conditioning should happen all day long, seven days a week, not just three times a week for a couple of sets of abdominal crunches. Think about this when you're working out, too. Abdominal conditioning should begin as soon as you walk into the gym and hop up onto the treadmill, the stair machine or the bike. You should be working your abdominals throughout your fitness class. You should be working your abdominals on every single exercise you do in the weight room. If you follow this type of prescription, you won't have to do hundreds of sit–ups. You'll be working your abdominals in a functional range while you're upright, instead of on your back. This is when we need our abdominals. When do we need our abs while we're on our back, anyway?

ABDOMINAL AND BACK EXERCISES

Here are some stabilization exercises that will get you not only looking better but also functioning better. Besides, our abdominals are more than just a fashion statement!

○ Heel Slide

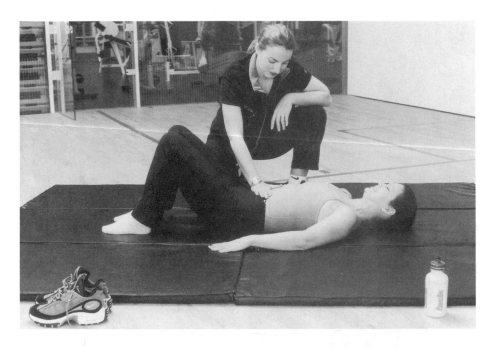

a. Take off your shoes. Lie on your back, with both legs bent and feet flat on the floor and slightly separated. Place your hands on your abdominals and contract them so that your abdominal cavity is concave (pulled inward). Stabilize your spine throughout the movement. Slowly slide one foot out on the floor until the leg is almost straight. Slowly slide it back into the starting position. Attempt the same movement with the opposite leg. Throughout the exercise, your two key reference points are that your abdominals must stay pulled inward and your vertebrae must not move. Your back should be completely stabilized and no arching or flexing of the spine should occur at any time.

b. If this exercise becomes easy, intensify the movement by sliding one leg out while the other leg is sliding in, so that both legs are moving simultaneously.

c. If this becomes easy, intensify the movement by sliding both legs out and in at the same time.

Perform any variation of the above exercises for 90 seconds.

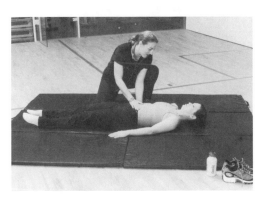

◎ Tripod

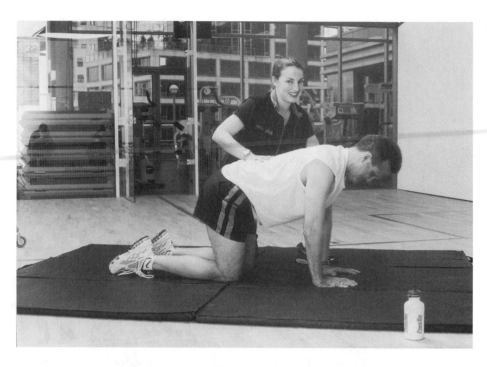

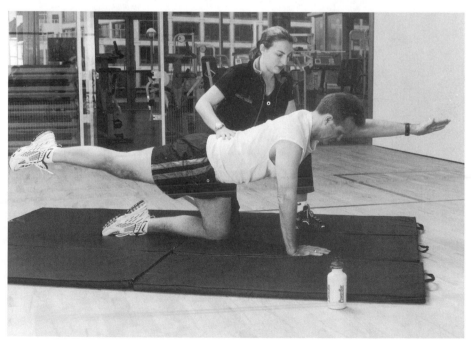

a. Start on your hands and knees with your arms directly under your shoulders and your knees directly underneath your hips. Keep your abdominals contracted inward and your spine completely stabilized. Your back should be totally neutral; it should feel as if there's a straight line from your tailbone to the top of your head. Your gaze should be down and slightly forward. Lift one arm, from the shoulder, and reach in front of you. Really stretch the arm forward and lift upward keeping your abdominals contracted and spine stabilized. Return to the starting position. Repeat the exercise, using the other arm. Perform the same movement with one leg. Then the other leg. While you lift one leg, be sure to not shift all your body weight to the side that is supporting you. Do this entire set 5 times.

b. If you want to intensify this movement, lift a diagonally opposed arm and leg at the same time. Do this 10 times on each side. Remember, the key reference points for this exercise are that you must keep the abdominals contracted inward and the back completely stabilized. Try to avoid arching your back as you lift your arms and/or legs. Think more about stretching out the arms and legs, than about lifting so high that you have to arch your back.

● Supine Bridge

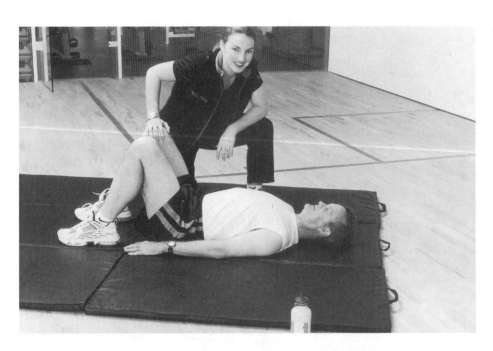

a. Lie on your back, with your knees bent and feet flat on the floor. Tighten your abdominal and buttock muscles and slowly lift your buttocks off the floor. Slowly roll up until your body weight is resting on the top of your shoulder blades and your knees and shoulders are in a straight line. Note: you are not resting on your neck but on your shoulder blades. Keep your hips square to the ceiling. Try to avoid letting your pelvis rotate. Hold this position for five seconds and then slowly release down. Perform 10 to 15 reps.

b. If you get strong enough, you can intensify this exercise by repeating the bridge position 10 to 15 times on one leg at a time.

○ Abdominal Alternating Leg Lift

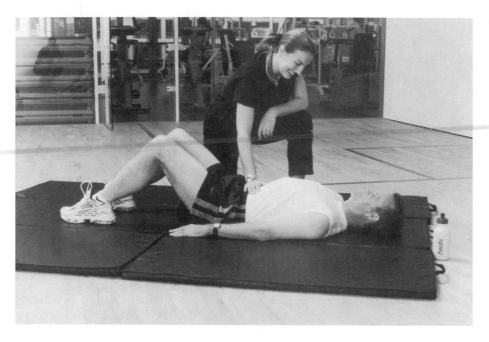

a. Lie on your back, with your knees bent and feet flat on the floor. Tighten your abdominal muscles and ensure that your low back is in a neutral, stabilized position. There should be no major space between your lower back and the floor and you should hold this position throughout the exercise. Slowly lift one leg off the floor a few inches and be sure that the movement of the leg occurs from the hip joint, not the knee joint. Perform 10 reps for each leg. Be sure that your back is stable throughout the exercise, so that there is no movement in the spine.

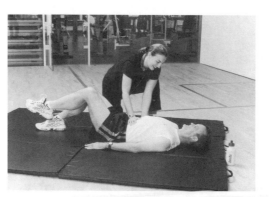

b. Once this becomes easy, do the same exercise with your legs straighter.

c. If you become really good you can try it with both legs at the same time, but keep your legs bent with this option. If you try this and your stomach muscles are pushing out and your back is arching, you're not working the right muscles and may be placing yourself at risk of injury.

⊙ Abdominal Alternating Leg Extension

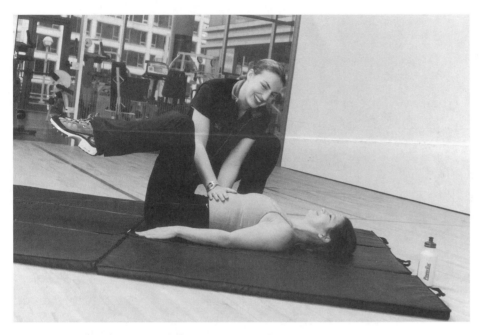

a. Lie on your back and lift your legs bent at the knee. Position your legs with a 90–degree angle at the knees and hips, so that your upper thighs are perpendicular to the floor and your lower legs are parallel to the floor. Tighten your abdominal muscles and stabilize your spine. Slowly extend one leg straight out to a 45–degree angle while the other leg remains still. Return the leg to the starting position and repeat with the other leg. Perform 10 reps for each leg.

b. If the exercise is too challenging, lower your leg to less than 45 degrees. If you want to intensify the movement, lower the leg closer to the floor, but remember your reference points at all times.

○ Abdominal Alternating Leg Lower

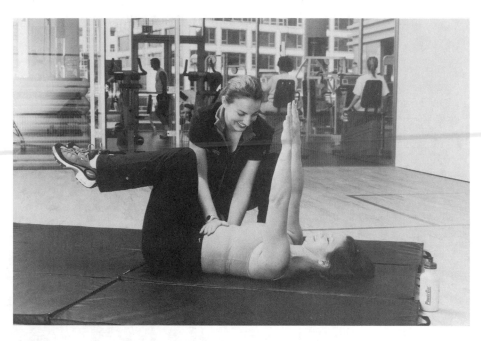

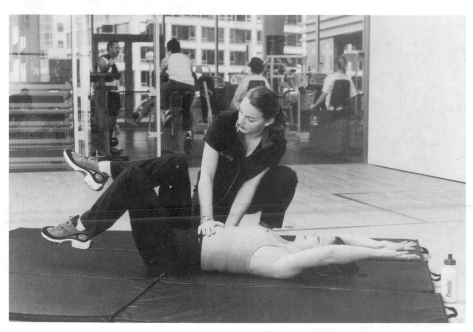

a. Lie on your back and lift your legs bent at the knee. Position your legs with a 90–degree angle at the knees and hips so that your upper thighs are perpendicular to the floor and your lower legs are parallel to the floor. Tighten your abdominal muscles and stabilize your spine. Keeping your knees at 90 degrees, slowly drop one heel toward the floor while the other leg remains still. Return the leg to the starting position and repeat with the other leg. Perform 10 reps for each leg.

b. If the exercise is too challenging, do not lower your leg all the way to the floor.

c. If you'd like to intensify the movement, you can add your arms. As one leg lowers to the ground, both arms also lower to the ground; as the leg lifts, both arms lift. In this option both the leg and arms are moving but the spine must remain stabilized.

○ Table Top

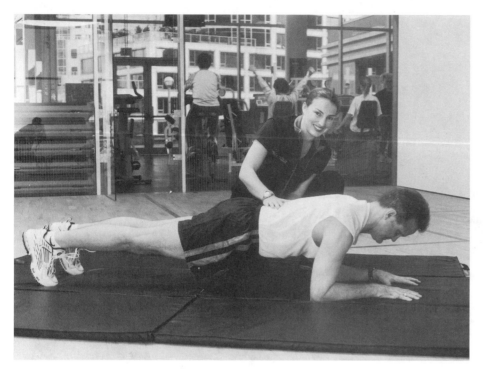

a. Lie on your stomach. Position your elbows under your shoulders. Contract your abdominal muscles and slowly lift your body onto your toes and elbows. Keep your back straight and shoulder blades pulled together. Remember to breathe. Hold this position for five seconds. Repeat 10 times.

b. This exercise is very intense, so I suggest you start by holding your body weight on your knees and elbows. As you get stronger, slowly progress to your toes.

○ Side Table Top

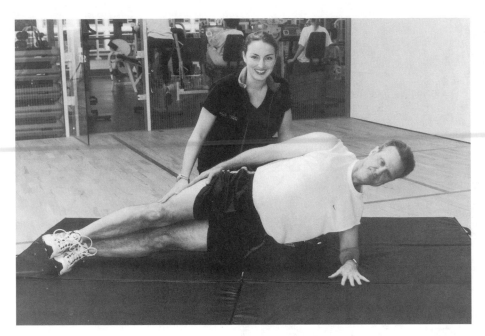

Lie on your side, with your legs straight. Position your elbows under your shoulders. Contract your abdominal muscles and slowly lift your body onto your feet and elbow. Keep your back straight. Remember to breathe. Hold this position for five seconds. Repeat 5 to 8 times on each side. You can also perform this exercise from your knees for a less advanced version.

⊙ Back Extension

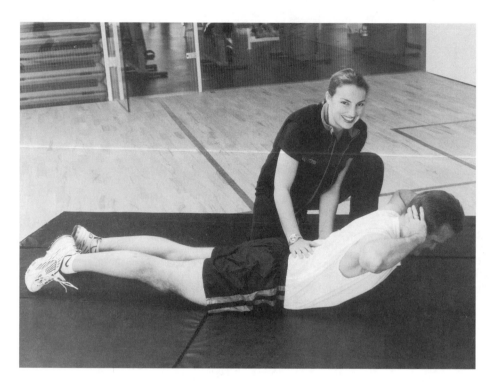

Lie on your stomach, with your hands behind your head and shoulder blades pulled together. Keep your stomach muscles contracted throughout the exercise. Slowly lift your chest off the floor. Hold for two or three seconds. Repeat 8 to 10 times.

○ Reverse Back Extension

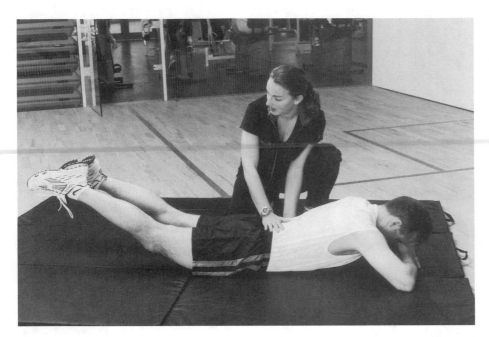

Lie on your stomach, with your head resting on your arms. Keep your abdominals contracted throughout the exercise. Slowly lift both legs off the floor. Hold for two to three seconds. Repeat 8 to 10 times.

Guidelines for Developing a Torso–Conditioning Program

When deciding which exercises to do and how often you'll perform them, follow these tips.

- Use a variety of exercises to ensure a balanced musculature.

- Use a variety of sequences. Mix up the order of the exercises.

- Spend more time on stabilization (as in the exercises just described) and less time on movement (crunches and sit–ups).

- Use a variety of contraction speeds. Use some fast and some slow movements.

- Use a variety of tools to add fun and diversity to your program (exercise balls, medicine balls, etc.).

- Use inclines and declines of benches to increase or decrease the intensity of movement or to ensure proper execution of movements.

- Train your torso muscles two to four times per week. The abdominal and back musculature is made up of striated, skeletal muscles. They're under voluntary control and behave just like any other muscle. Therefore, the work:rest training ratio principles are similar to any other muscle group. You do not need to train your abs every day to get results. If you commit to your submaximal daily abdominal contractions, performing some of the listed exercises a couple of times a week will do the trick.

- Work up to one set of 20 reps of the exercises.

- Remember that spot reduction is a myth. Abdominal exercises do not get rid of fat from your abdominal region. There is no direct metabolic pathway from the muscle cells in your abdominal area to the fat cells surrounding them. For any muscle to use stored fat for energy, your body must first send the stored fat to the liver. The liver converts this fat into fatty acids and then sends it to the muscles to be used as fuel. Unfortunately, the fat that the abdominal muscles uses may not be from the fat in the abdominal region; the energy to perform an abdominal exercise may come from fat stores in your arms. Localized fat mobilization is dependent on genetics. The key to reducing fat in and around your stomach is a program that includes regular cardiovascular exercise, muscle–conditioning exercise and good nutrition — and, of course, patience! However, performing many of the stabilization exercises listed here will increase your ability to hold your abdominal cavity inward and will give you the appearance of a smaller waist.

SHOULDER EXERCISES

Anyone who has experienced a shoulder injury can attest that it can cause excruciating pain affecting one's daily life. The shoulder joint is a relatively unstable structure of muscles, tendons and ligaments. It provides great range of motion, but to achieve this mobility it sacrifices stability, making it more susceptible to injury. Popular sports such as swimming, baseball and racquet sports require repetitive movement that can present a high risk of shoulder injury. Aging brings on changes that put us at further risk of shoulder pain.

One common complaint is the rotator cuff tear. The rotator cuff is a group of four muscles in the shoulder region. Pain can result from tears in any one of the rotator cuff tendons (where the cuff muscles attach to the bone). As we age, these tendons become weaker and the risk of tearing increases.

Another example is an impinged shoulder, which can result from a shrinking of the subacromion space between the shoulder blade, collarbone and upper arm. As we get older this space in our shoulder joint gets smaller and smaller, increasing the chances of nerves being. Impingement can be extremely painful, affecting an individual's ability to lift and carry and perform day–to–day activities.

Since none of us can fully escape the effects of aging, we're all at risk. Here are some exercises you can start doing immediately to help reduce the danger later.

○ Prone Retraction & Arm Lift

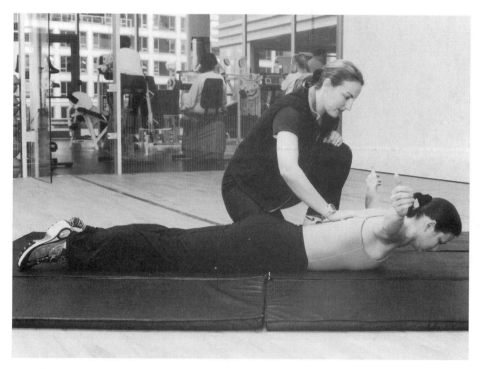

a. Lying on your stomach, stretch your arms straight out to the sides. Turn your thumbs up to the ceiling, then slowly lift your arms. Concentrate on pulling your shoulder blades together. Be sure to avoid pressing your arms backwards — they should be moving up, not back. You may want to put a towel under your head to keep your neck in a neutral position. Do 8 to 15 reps.

b. Do as above, but this time extend your arms in front of you on the floor, instead of out to the sides — thumbs are still up. Lift both arms 8 to 15 times.

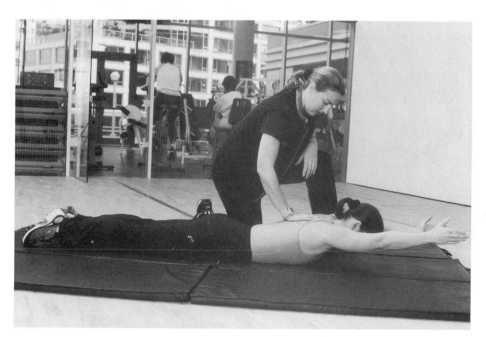

○ Supine Back Press

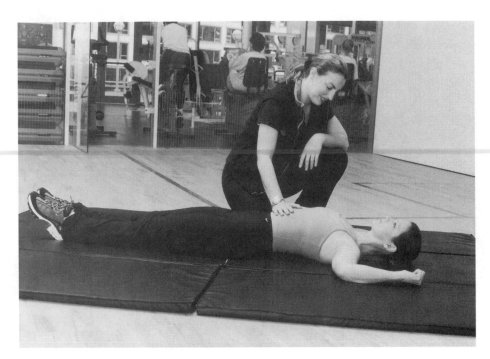

Lie on your back, with your arms overhead and your elbow and shoulder joints at 90–degrees in a "Hands up!" position. Press your elbows and the backs of your wrists into the floor. Hold for five seconds. Repeat 8 to 15 times.

○ Pendulum Stretch

Grab two cans of food or two dumbbells. Stand tall, let your arms hang by your sides with your palms facing into your body. Relax your shoulders and let your arms dangle. Perform small circles in both directions for one minute each.

○ "Hands Up!"

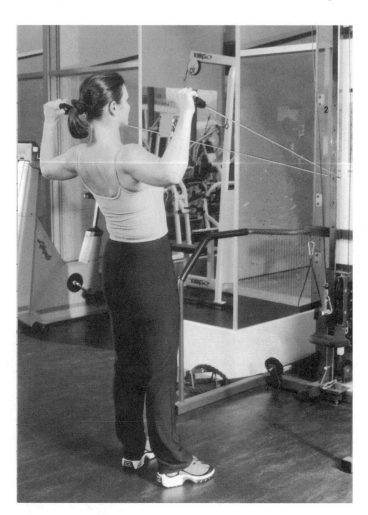

Wrap a tube around a pole and hold one end of the tube in each hand. Start with your arms outstretched in front of your body, with your palms down. Slowly lift your arms backwards until they finish in the "Hands up!" position. Do 8 to 15 reps.

○ External Rotation

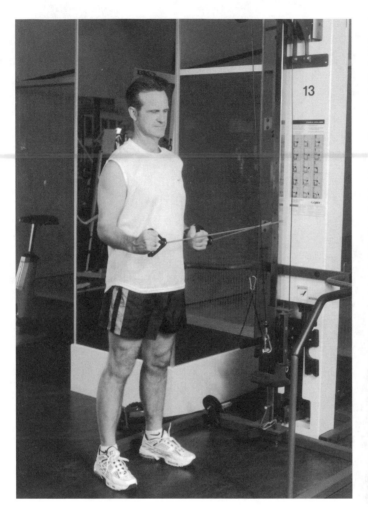

Wrap a tube around a pole and position it so that it is at elbow height. Start by standing sideways to the pole. The inside arm is just holding onto one end of the tube. The outside arm is holding the other end with the elbow at a 90–degree angle and positioned right beside the waist. With your palm facing the pulley, keep your upper arm completely still and your elbow at your side. Slowly rotate your forearm out and away from your body. Return to the starting position. Repeat 8 to 15 times for each arm.

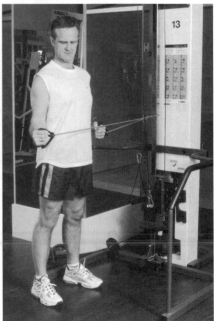

KNEE EXERCISES

Many knee injuries occur as a result of muscular imbalances in the lower body. Your knee joint is composed of the long bone of the thigh, the femur, articulating over the smaller shinbone, the tibia. The patella, or kneecap, slides through a small groove as your knee bends and straightens. If there are any muscular imbalances in your front thigh muscles, your quadriceps pull the kneecap either to the left or right of the groove, causing the kneecap to track less smoothly. The articulation may become a more damaging movement, eventually causing pain. Years and years of this type of misalignment will cause degeneration and wear and tear that will lead to pain that can dramatically affect your life.

Here are some exercises to help strengthen the muscles surrounding the joint and teach your knees proper tracking.

○ Knee Dips

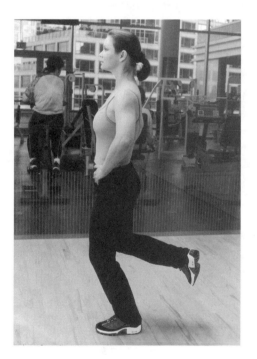

Stand in front of a mirror. Point your toes straight forward. Square your hips and shoulders to the mirror, so that you are facing straight into it. Imagine that you have a string attached to the top of your head and it's pulling your body straight up so that your posture is perfect. Lift one leg and balance on the other. Look into the mirror at the knee of the supporting leg and make sure it points straight forward. Avoid leaning into the hip of the supporting leg. Slowly bend your supporting leg, lowering your body weight down and up only a few inches. Your primary focus is to ensure that your kneecap doesn't collapse in toward the midline of your body and that you're not leaning into your hips. Make sure your knee is not wobbling but is, completely stabilized. Do 8 to 15 reps for each leg.

HAMSTRING EXERCISES

Another common imbalance arises when the front thigh muscles, the quadriceps, are significantly stronger than the back thigh muscles, the hamstrings. This can increase the risk of knee problems. You learned hamstring curls and related exercises in the muscle conditioning section and also a supine bridging exercise in the abdominal section of this subsection, which are all excellent for hamstrings. Here's another of my favorites.

○ Ball Hamstring Curls

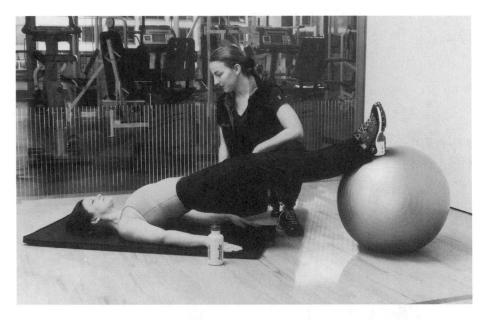

Lie on your back, with your feet positioned on an exercise ball. With your arms at your sides, slowly lift your hips and buttocks toward the ceiling while contracting your buttocks and hamstrings, until your body weight is resting comfortably on your shoulder blades. Throughout the exercise, be sure to keep your hips square to the ceiling and your abdominals contracted. Slowly, bending your knees, curl the ball in toward your body while maintaining control and stability through your core area. Slowly curl out and in. Repeat eight to 15 times.

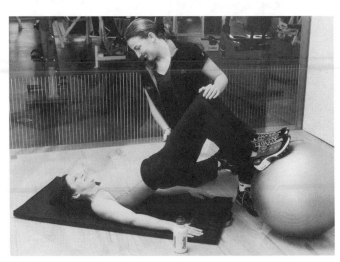

You now have a variety of tools to help you keep your back, knees and shoulders strong and healthy as you age. And, of course, your abs are going to look marvelous!

Balance Training

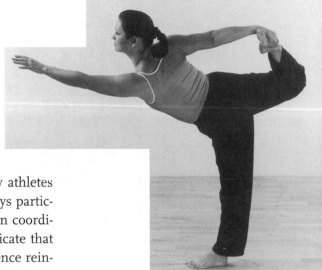

Falls and impaired mobility are a serious problem for our aging population. The good news is that much of the decline in balance can be reversed through a program of balance training. One study found that healthy people as old as 90 can reduce the tendency to fall by 50 per cent. It's not hard to see that this can help keep people independent and mobile far longer, as well as reduce their risk of injury.

Balance is an integral component of almost all sports, yet many athletes neglect this aspect of their training. An athlete, older or not, who pays particular attention to balance conditioning will notice an improvement in coordination and in ability to transfer strength to movement. Studies indicate that athletes who have suffered from an injury are more likely to experience reinjury. This recurrence can be linked to failure to incorporate balance training into rehab programs.

Today, injury rehabilitation almost always includes a number of different balance exercises to ensure the patient develops kinesthetic body awareness — the body's ability to find and maintain neutral and effective alignment in the affected joint. This helps restore the previous level of coordination, agility, strength and endurance. Balance training is absolutely critical for restoring normal functioning of joints and muscles. Without balance training, the healing joints and muscles are not as proficient at staying in their neutral, safe positions and may function inappropriately under unforeseen conditions, thus causing reinjury.

You don't need a tightrope to train your balance system. Here's a variety of exercises to help you implement this type of training into your workouts.

◎ One–legged Stance

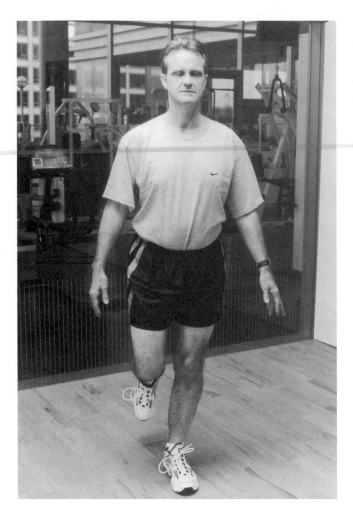

Begin by standing on one foot, with fully upright posture. Hold for 30 seconds, each side. Once you're able to hold your balance without obbling, do this exercise with your eyes closed. If your balance isn't very good to begin with, you may want to have something sturdy close by to steady you if you waver.

Upper Body & One–legged Stance

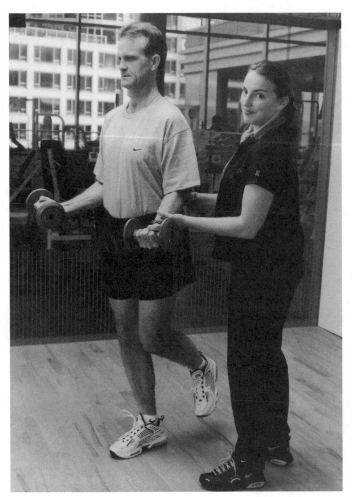

It's easy to implement balance training while doing traditional upper body exercises. Do on one leg any exercise that you would generally do standing on both legs.

2 × 4 Training

Head down to your local hardware store and pick up a long piece of 2" x 4" lumber. You can walk along the wood as if you are on a tightrope, then do the same on your toes, and then try it walking backwards. You can step sideways up and down the timber. You can throw a ball to and catch a ball from a partner while maintaining balance on the 2" x 4". Your options are endless. You can also do these exercises along a curb or on a log at the beach or park.

Exercise Balls

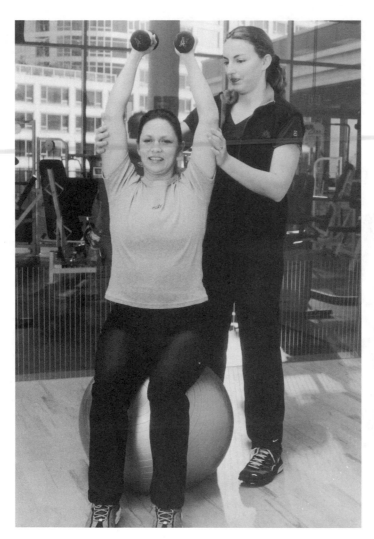

Any exercise you do sitting or lying on a bench can be advanced by incorporating an exercise ball. By sitting on the ball and performing, say, an overhead shoulder press, your stabilizing muscles have to work much harder because you are positioned on an unstable piece of apparatus. The same goes for lying over the exercise ball and performing, say, a chest press. By lying on the ball instead of a bench your stabilizing muscles are challenged to a greater degree.

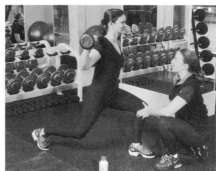

○ Wobble Boards

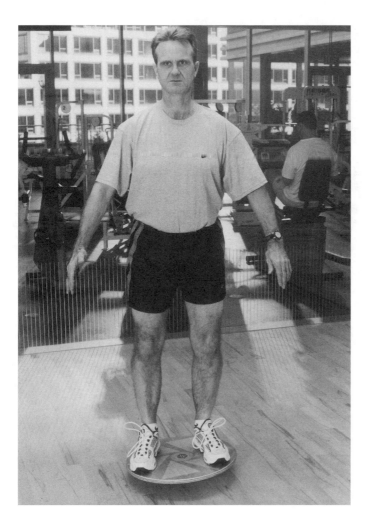

There are various models of wobble boards, from less to more advanced versions. You can attempt to balance on one or two legs. Make it a game and see how long you can balance before an edge touches down. Maintain perfect posture, and remember to stand close to something sturdy until you get good at these exercises. Once you master the wobble board, you can continue to challenge yourself with it by performing other activities such as bicep curls or catching and throwing a ball while balancing.

○ Pro Fitter

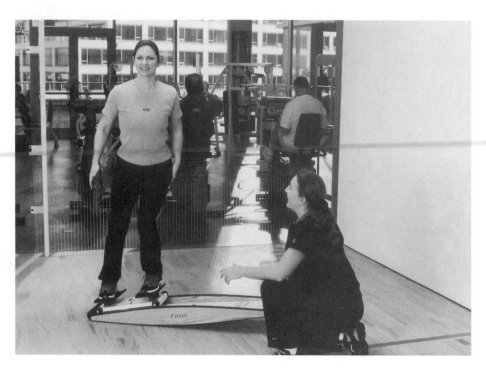

This is an excellent tool for developing balance. You stand on a moveable platform that slides you from side to side or forward and backwards. This piece of equipment comes with a video and a booklet that demonstrates a variety of balance and muscle–conditioning exercises for the entire body. As you can imagine it is a great conditioning tool for any level of skier, whether on water or snow.

○ Foam Rollers

These are made of foam and are long and cylindrical. You can attempt to stand on them, perform squats and lunges on them, or complete abdominal stabilization exercises while lying on them.

Fitter International also sells exercise balls and other balance products. Take a few of these exercises and perform them a couple of times per week. Soon you'll be in balance.

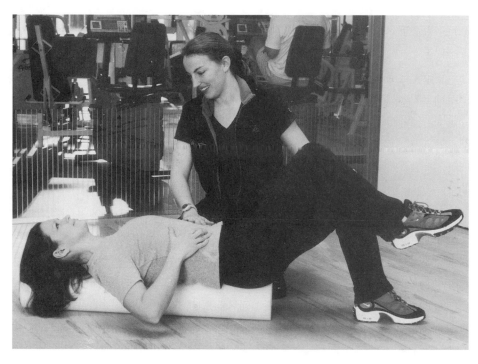

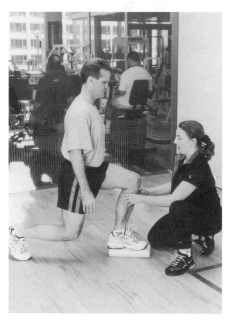

For those of you who are more serious about developing your balance, there are a number of balance products available. Fitter International (1–800–FIT-TER1; www.fitter1.com), a company based in Calgary, Alberta, Canada, specializes in balance products. Here's a look at what it offers, though you will find similar equipment at other outlets, too.

SPORTS

There are some sports that will condition your balance without your even having to think about it. Ice–skating, in–line skating, alpine skiing, snowboarding and waterskiing are among the sports that will maintain high levels of balance as you age.

Flexibility Training

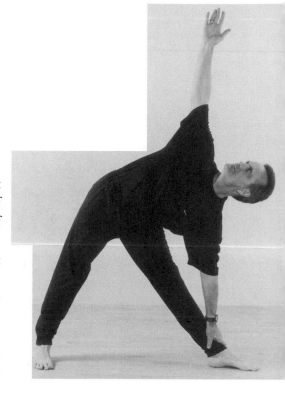

As we age, our connective tissue becomes more and more rigid. If we're tight to begin with, this is really going to affect our posture, alignment and risk of injury. Add to this the fact that stretching is the most neglected component of fitness and we've got a problem.

Most people either don't stretch correctly or for long enough or they skip it all together.

Unfortunately, those who neglect stretching are almost always those who need it the most. The people who take the time to stretch are usually the ones who are really good at it. You can find them in front of a mirror in a full straddle position, with their chests to the floor, or in an all–out hamstring stretch with their legs positioned almost behind their heads! They enjoy stretching because it feels so good to them.

But for people who are tight, stretching is usually a painful experience. Their muscles shake and they can't wait to release the stretch. Typically, their posture is terrible as they're holding the stretch. It's easy to see why they eliminate stretching from their workout.

After working in the fitness industry for more than a decade I've finally come up with a system that has even my most rigid, tight, can't–touch–my–toes clients enjoying their stretching segments. I've found that if I can make a stretch comfortable enough that clients don't even realize they're stretching, they will often hold it long enough to allow the muscles to lengthen.

The following wall stretches are the most successful in increasing enjoyment of the stretching segment. While my clients are stretching, their backs are in a neutral position that is very comfortable. They don't have to use any of their muscles to support their backs. They can just relax and focus on the stretch. They can also read or watch TV in this position, which may increase the amount of time they hold any stretch. My clients are finding these stretching segments so enjoyable that they're holding stretches longer than they have before and are now stretching every day. They would never have dreamed of stretching this much before.

Keep this in mind: Regular flexibility training can reduce common aches and pains associated with aging and various forms of arthritis, reduce your risk of injury and help improve your posture and functioning.

"Exercise, exercise your powers; what is difficult will finally become routine."
—George C. Lichtenberg

○ Hamstrings

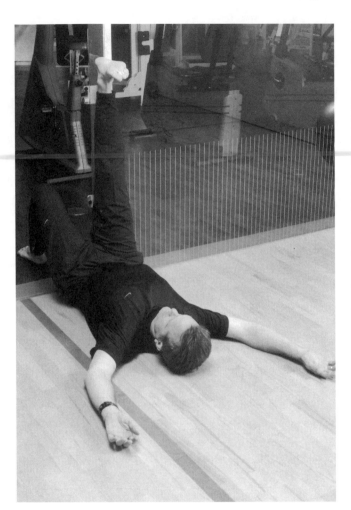

Lie on your back in an open doorway and position one leg on the wall, with your heel toward the ceiling. The other leg should be bent, with your foot on the floor. Find a position where you can feel a light stretch in the back of your thigh. To make the stretch more intense, move your buttocks closer to the wall; to make it less intense, move your buttocks farther from the wall. Hold this stretch for as long as you feel comfortable — a minimum of 30 seconds for each leg but ideally longer. Try to relax and breathe into the stretch. Feel free to read a magazine or watch TV while holding this stretch

○ Groin

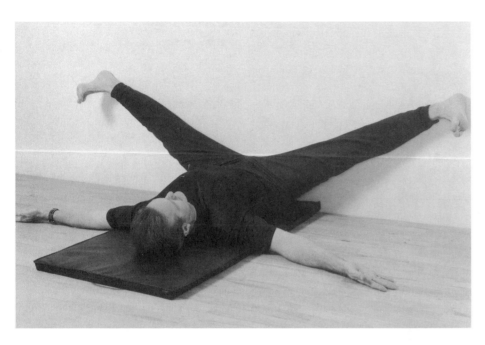

a. Lie on your back, with both legs straight up against a wall. Slowly separate your legs into a V position until you feel a light stretch through your groin area. Hold for a minimum of 30 seconds. Feel free to hold longer.

b. Sit with your back pressed against a wall. Bring the soles of your feet together and let your knees drop toward the floor. Maintain perfect upright posture. Hold for 30 seconds or longer.

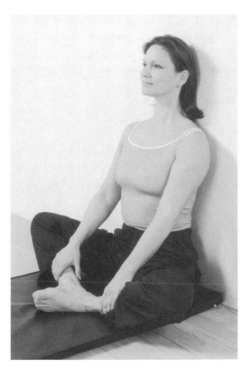

◎ Hips & Back

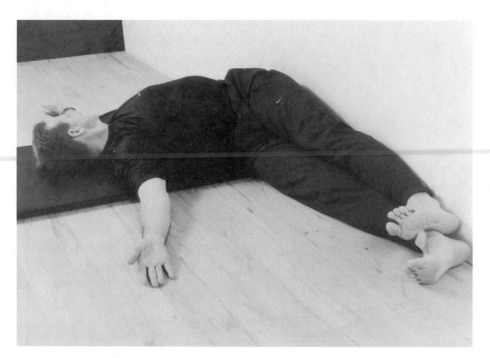

Lie on your back, with both legs straight up against a wall. Slowly let both legs fall to one side. Try to feel this stretch through your hips and lightly through your back. To intensify the stretch, move the top leg a few inches away from the wall but keep it straight. Hold for 30 seconds or longer, on each side.

⊙ Glutes

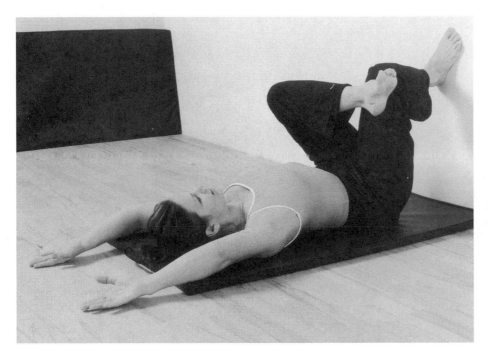

Lie on your back, with your buttocks about a foot away from a wall. Position one leg so that the bottom of the foot is in contact with the wall and the knee is at 90–degrees. Cross the other leg over so that the ankle is resting on the thigh. To make the stretch less intense, move your buttocks farther from the wall; to make it more intense, move your buttocks closer to the wall or lightly press the crossed leg toward the wall. Hold for 30 seconds or longer, on each side.

Here are some other important stretches to help reverse the aging process.

⊙ Quadricep

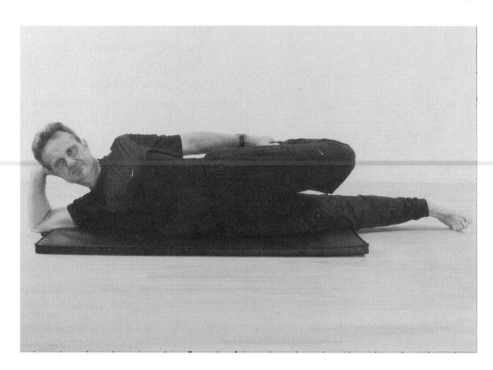

Lie on your side, with your body straight. Bend the top knee and bring your foot toward your buttock so that you can grab your foot or ankle. Hold the stretch while pressing your hip forward and your knee slightly back. Hold for 30 seconds or longer, each side.

⊙ Hip Flexor

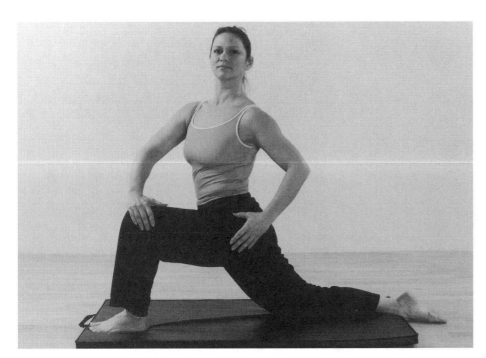

Position yourself in a lunge position, with your front knee over the front ankle and your back knee comfortably on a mat or towel. Straighten your spine so that your posture is fully erect. Lightly press the back hip forward. Feel the stretch in the front of this thigh. To intensify the stretch, keep your body tall while you turn your upper body in toward your front knee. Hold for 30 seconds or longer, on each side.

○ Calf

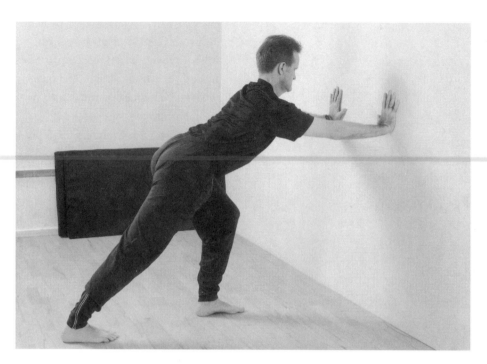

Stand facing a wall. Place one leg close to the wall and the other farther away. Keep the heel of the back leg firmly on the floor. Be sure that both feet face forward. Feel the stretch in the back calf. Hold for 30 seconds or longer. Now move the back foot in a few inches. Keep it firmly planted on the ground, but slightly bend the back knee and hold the stretch. Hold for 30 seconds or longer, on each side.

○ Ball Stretch

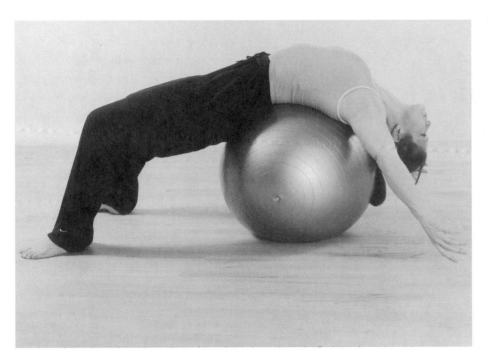

This is one of my favorite passive stretches to help someone improve common postural deviations. Sit on an exercise ball. Slowly walk your feet forward until you are lying over the ball; your hips, back and shoulders should round back over the ball. Place your arms to the sides of your body and hold this position. Then extend your hands over your head and hold this position. Your head should be supported on the ball throughout the sequence. I like to hold this stretch for a long time, especially after a long day over the computer.

Remember to hold each stretch for at least 30 seconds. This is when the real stretching begins, so holding a stretch for anything less than 30 seconds is not going to increase your flexibility. Remember that light stretching is much better than deep, painful stretching. It's also very important to note that deep stretching should take place after your workouts are otherwise complete, when your muscles are warm and most pliable.

Another great way to improve your flexibility is to enroll in a yoga or Pilates–based program, which incorporates a high degree of flexibility training.

YOGA
Here are a few yogic poses that you can try on your own.

◎ Dancer's Pose

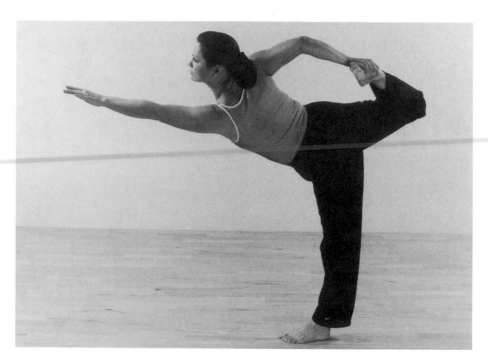

Lift your right leg behind you, finding a good balance on your left leg. Gently take hold of the right foot with your right hand. Move the right leg farther back while tilting the body forward, with your left arm stretched above your head. Bend your upper body as far forward as feels comfortable. Hold for five breaths. Repeat with the other leg.

○ Airplane Pose

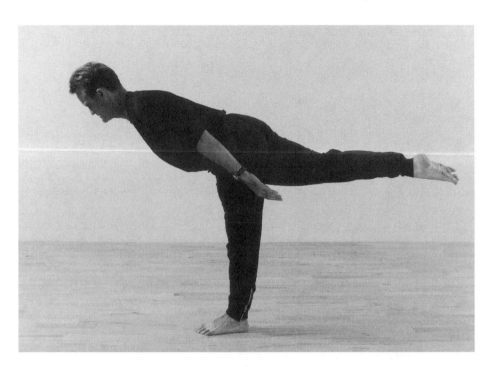

With arms at your sides, fingers stretched outward, slowly bend your upper body until it is parallel with the floor (or as low as feels comfortable) as you lift one leg behind you. Keep your raised leg and dropped arms very straight, stretching out long and strong. Be sure to keep your hips squared — do not let one hip rise higher than the other. Hold for five breaths. Repeat with the other leg.

⊙ Lightning Bolt Pose

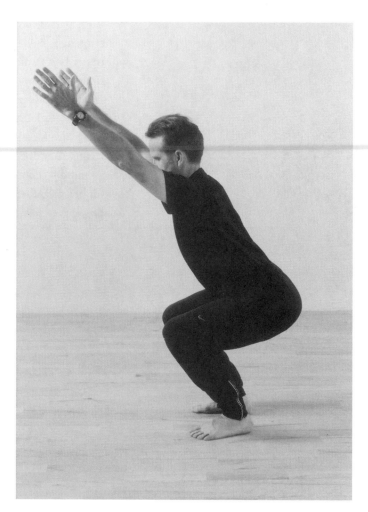

Stand with your feet together, eyes gazing straight ahead. Exhale, bend your knees and lift your arms overhead, with palms together. Your extended arms should be in line with your torso. Breathe deeply. When you inhale, return to the standing position. Repeat 5 times.

○ Warrior One Pose

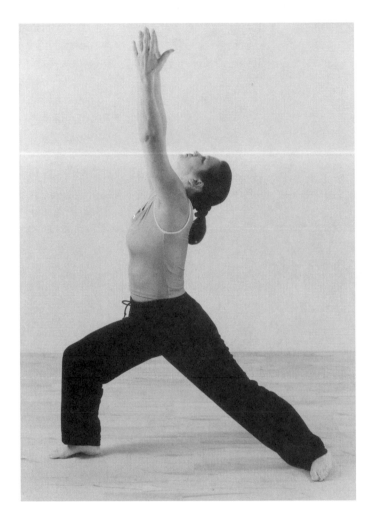

Standing in a lunge position, place one foot in front of the other as if walking on a tightrope. Turn the back foot outward on a diagonal. Keep the front knee above the ankle and your hips and shoulders facing toward the front knee. Extend the arms upward and reach toward the ceiling. Hold for five breaths. Repeat on the other side.

○ Triangle Pose

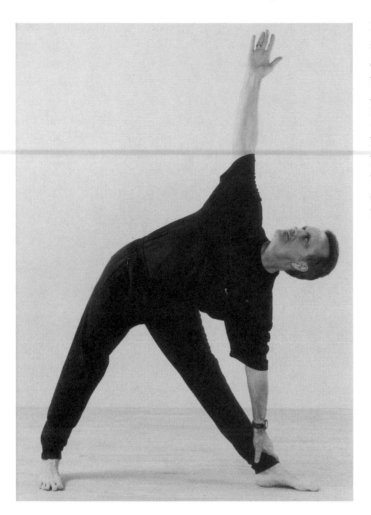

Position your legs wider apart than shoulder width. Turn the left foot outward, directly to the side. Keep both legs straight as you slowly drop your left arm to touch your foot. Reach the right arm straight up as you look to the ceiling. Imagine that you are wedged between two walls so that all your body parts are lined up on the same plane. Hold for five breaths. Repeat on the other side.

○ Forward Bend Pose

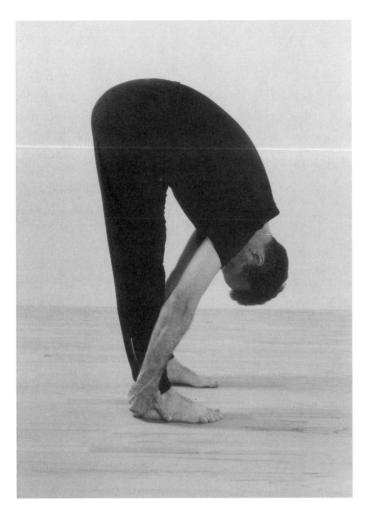

Stand with your hands along the sides of your body. Slowly bring your hands toward the floor by bending at the waist, without bending your knees. Place both hands behind your calves. Relax your neck. For a further stretch, place your hands by the sides of your feet, with the fingers pointing forward. Hold for five breaths. Repeat 3 to 5 times.

⊙ Tree Pose

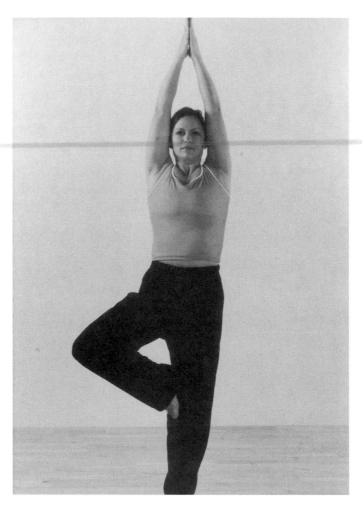

Stand on one leg. Lift the other leg and place its foot as high as you can on the inner thigh of the extended leg, with your toes pointing toward the floor. Raise your arms above your head, press your shoulders down and extend your fingers upward. Keep your hips square, press your bent knee toward the back wall and make sure your tailbone stays down. Hold for five breaths. Repeat on the other side.

○ Cat Tilt Pose

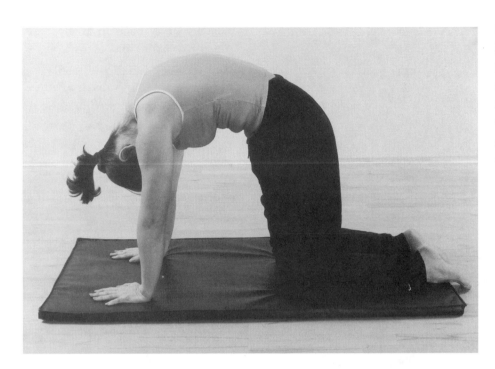

Start on the floor on your elbows and knees. Contract your abdominals and round your back, letting your head drop toward the floor. Return to neutral. Arch your back, looking up to the ceiling. Remember to move slowly and breathe into each phase of the movement. Repeat 3 to 5 times.

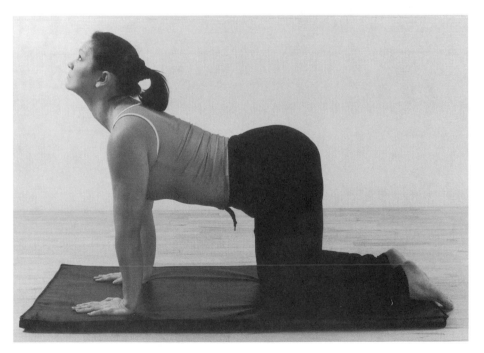

○ Upward–Dog Pose

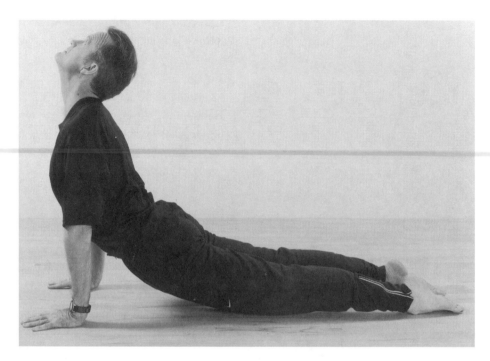

Lie on your stomach on the floor. Place your hands shoulder width apart, with fingers pointing forward. Slowly extend your arms, lifting the chest up and out and rolling your shoulders back. Press down on the tops of the feet and engage the thighs and hips to lift the thighs off the floor. Hold for five breaths. Repeat 3 to 5 times.

○ Plank Pose

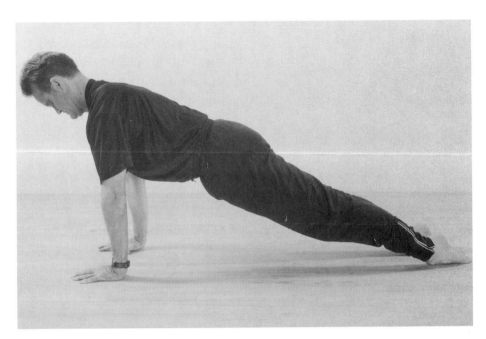

From the upward–dog position, lift your thighs right off the floor so that there is a straight line from your neck to your toes. Hold for five breaths. Repeat 3 to 5 times.

⊙ Downward-Facing Dog Pose

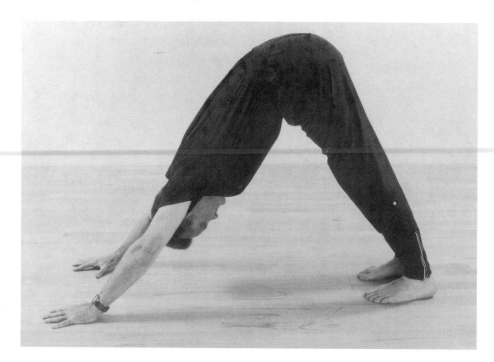

From the plank position, lift your hips toward the ceiling and press your heels to the floor. There should be a straight line from your hands to your hips. Hold for five breaths. Repeat 3 to 5 times.

PILATES

Pilates is a 90–year–old exercise discipline named for Joseph Pilates and once popular only among dancers, actresses and gymnasts. Today, average exercisers, athletes and those suffering from an injury are experiencing the benefits. It is noted for improving your posture and alignment, producing long, lean muscles and improving your core abdominal strength. If you'd like more information about Pilates or would like to purchase Pilates–based videos, contact Stott Pilates, a Canadian company at 1–800–910–0001, or visit its website at **www.stottpilates.com**

Nutrition

There is no trick to eating well to help you slow the aging process. It's stuff we have all heard before. Drink lots of water. Consume your required intake of fruits, vegetables and whole–grain products. Minimize fat, alcohol and sugar intake. But there seems to be a gap between knowing what to do and actually adhering to these simple guidelines. There is no special grapefruit, cabbage, low–protein or high–protein diet or pill that will get you the results you want quickly. Knowledge alone is not power. We all know what we have to do!

It is finding the motivation and inspiration to make and adhere to very small changes in our nutrition plan that will bring success. Finding the motivation to stick to a healthy nutrition plan day–in, day–out is all it takes. Here's the good news: you don't have to starve yourself, and you don't have to limit your diet to carrots and broccoli.

Very small changes to your eating habits will often bring about big differences. The new habits just need to be consistent and ongoing. Perhaps start with one area at a time. Once you have that habit mastered, tackle the next nutrition goal. By taking one step at a time, soon your diet will provide you with all the nutrients necessary to slow the aging process.

Health Problem	Nutrient	Amount	Recommendations
Breast cancer	Dietary fat	Too much	Reduce intake to less than 30% of total calories.
	Alcohol	Too much	Consume alcohol in moderation, if at all.
Colon cancer	Dietary fat	Too much	Increase complete carbohydrates (4–6 servings of grains, 2–4 fruits, 3–5 servings of vegetables/day).
	Dietary fiber	Too little	Increase fiber in diet (4–6 servings of grains, 2–4 fruits, 3–5 servings of vegetables/day).
Heart disease	Saturated fat	Too much	Reduce dietary saturated fat intake to less than 8% of total calories.
	Cholesterol	Too much	Reduce dietary cholesterol to less than 300mg/day.
	Dietary fiber	Too little	Increase complex carbohydrates and dietary fiber intake.
High blood pressure	Salt	Too much	Reduce dietary salt/sodium intake by not adding table salt and limiting intake of processed foods.
	Alcohol	Too much	Consume alcohol in moderation, if at all.
	Calcium	Too little	Increase nonfat or low–fat milk/milk product intake.
Liver disease	Alcohol	Too much	Consume alcohol in moderation, if at all.
Lung cancer	Beta–carotene	Too little	Increase dietary intake of fruits and vegetables, especially oranges, yellows and dark greens.
Osteoporosis	Calcium	Too little	Increase calcium intake to two servings of fat–free or low–fat milk or milk products/day.
	Protein	Too much	Consume only moderate amounts of protein (0.8–1.2g/kg/body weight/day).
Stress	Caffeine	Too much	Reduce intake of foods and beverages containing caffeine or switch to decaffeinated products.

Adapted from Williams, M.H. 1995. Nutrition for Fitness & Sport, 4th Edition. Dubuque, IA: Brown & Benchmark as seen in Kasdan, T. S., 1997. A Recipe for Aging. IDEA Today November/December 1997: 33–41.

Here are a few antiaging nutrition habits you might like to develop.

Antiaging Nutrition Habit #1

Consume a balanced diet that is rich in fiber. Ensure your diet is 60 to 65 per cent carbohydrate content — that is, fruits, vegetables, breads, pastas and rice. Of this amount, 55 per cent should be in the form of complex carbohydrates and whole–grain products, and no more than 10 per cent from simple carbo- hydrates (cakes, etc.). Complement this with a diet that is 20 to 30 per cent fat content, and finally balance off your diet with 15 per cent protein content — that is, meats, soy and dairy products. It is important to note that, although protein deficiency plays a role in the development of osteoporosis, too much protein can also promote bone loss. So it is imperative to get the correct amount of protein and avoid eating protein in excess.

This type of balanced diet will help you maintain a healthy body composi- tion and weight and provide you with the nutrients for optimal health and functioning.

Due to the increased risk of osteoporosis as we age, we should be consum- ing a minimum of two servings of fat–free or low–fat milk or milk products every day. This will provide the required amounts of calcium and an excellent source of protein, riboflavin and other nutrients. Most milk is fortified with vitamin D, and vitamin A is added back into skim milk to replace nutrients lost when fat is removed. Keep in mind, however, that if you suffer from lac- tose intolerance that causes gas, bloating or diarrhea you may have to find a different source for these compounds. Luckily, most markets now sell nonfat and one per cent lactose–free (predigested lactose) milk and cottage cheese. Other foods (e.g., tofu and calcium–fortified soy drinks, broccoli) can also pro- vide calcium.

As you begin to reduce the amount of fat and increase the amount of fruits, vegetables and whole–grain products in your diet, your fiber intake will auto- matically increase. But as you start to adopt these healthy habits, you may notice that you experience more intestinal gas. To reduce the initial negative effects of a high–fiber diet, change your diet gradually and soon your body will adapt. You might also consider taking an anti-gas product that will help you manage these side effects.

Those aged 60 and older should try to get the recommended 20 to 35 grams of fiber each day by consuming a minimum of two servings of fruit, three serv- ings of vegetables and four servings of whole–grains. But you should avoid increasing your fiber intake to greater amounts than these listed, because too much fiber can exacerbate existing impairment of the gastrointestinal tract. You might choose to avoid spicy foods if you suffer from gastrointestinal prob- lems, and this may also help prevent hot flashes.

> "Some people never seem to grow old. Always active in thought, always ready to adopt new ideas, they are never chargeable to fogeyism. Satisfied, yet ever dissatisfied, settled, yet ever unsettled, they always enjoy the best of what is, and are the first to find the best of what will be…"
>
> —WILLIAM SHAKESPEARE

When I say "balanced," I really mean balanced. That is, all foods can be eaten in a healthy diet. You just need to have some boundaries and parameters. I prefer to follow the 80:20 rule for nutrition, which holds that if you are eating well 80 per cent of the time, you can allow yourself to indulge in the other 20 per cent. Eating well 80 per cent of the time will definitely keep you healthy and will be a much more enjoyable process. This type of belief system is focused on the long term, so if you adopt it it's important that you decide to do only things that you can see yourself doing for the rest of your days. The only way to achieve your goals is to disrupt your life as little as possible so that you're less likely to be disheartened and fail.

If you follow a balanced diet, you should have no problem obtaining the recommended daily allowances (RDA). Here is a chart listing the essential vitamins and minerals to help reverse the aging process, and foods in which they can be found.

Vitamin/Mineral	Benefits	Common Food Sources
Vitamin A RDA = 5,000 IU for men RDA = 4,000 IU for women	Helps maintain vision, skin, hair, gums, mucus membranes; acts as antioxidant, protecting cells from free radicals.	Liver, fish oil, fortified milk.
Beta–carotene No RDA	Reduces risk of cancer, heart disease.	Orange, yellow, red, dark green fruits/vegetables.
Vitamin B12 RDA = 2 micrograms	Coenzyme for formation of DNA, including DNA that develops red blood cells. Deficiency in vitamin B12 can lead to pernicious (deadly) anemia.	Found in animal products: meat, fish, poultry, dairy, eggs
Vitamin C RDA = 60 mg	Antioxidant that promotes healing, fights infection, metabolizes amino acids, increases iron absorption.	Citrus fruits, dark green vegetables, potatoes. RDA = 1 citrus fruit and 170 mL of citrus fruit juice.
Vitamin D RDA = 5 micrograms	Helps build bones and teeth and maintain calcium and phosphorus levels in blood.	Eggs, fatty fish, liver; synthetically in fortified milk and milk products; 10–20 minutes of sunshine two or three times a week converts a provitamin in skin into normal blood levels of vitamin D.

Vitamin E RDA = 10 mg for women RDA = 8 mg for women	Antioxidant that protects body from free radicals. Widely touted as having the capacity to reduce signs and symptoms of aging.	Poultry, seafood, seeds, nuts, dark green vegetables, wheat germ, fortified cereals, eggs.
Calcium RDA = 1,000 mg Postmenopausal women, and older men may benefit from 1,000–1,500 mg Estrogen–deficient women may benefit from 1,500 mg	Essential to bone formation, nerve impulse transmission, muscle contraction, enzyme activation of vitamin B12.	Dairy products, legumes, dark green vegetables, calcium–fortified juices.
Iron RDA = 10 mg	Aids in transport and activation of oxygen.	Meat, fish, poultry, legumes, dark green vegetables, dried fruits, fortified cereals. Heme iron, found in animal protein, is about 15% absorbable; nonheme iron, found in vegetable protein, is only 3–5% absorbable. Nonheme iron absorption can be increased by using cast–iron cookware, consuming a source of vitamin C with meals; avoiding tea and coffee.
Manganese No RDA	Works with copper and zinc to build bone.	Red meat.
Phosphorus RDA = 800 mg	Helps build bones.	Dairy products, meat, fish, poultry, legumes, grains.
Sodium Limit to less than 2,000 mg each day	Decrease intake of sodium to control high blood pressure and reduce water retention.	Table salt; cheese; pickled foods; fast foods; canned, prepared, frozen foods; some condiments; snack foods.
Potassium	May be beneficial for high blood pressure.	Bananas, oranges, cantaloupe, tomatoes, potatoes, dried figs, beans.
Zinc RDA = 15 mg for men RDA = 12 mg for women	Cofactor of many enzymes involved in energy metabolism, wound healing, immune response.	Meat, fish, poultry, dairy products, whole–grains, dark green vegetables.

Adapted from Kasdan, T.S., 1997. "A Recipe for Aging." IDEA Today, November/December 1997: 33–41.
RDA = recommended daily allowance

Antiaging Nutrition Habit #2

Drink more water. Did you know that 50 to 60 per cent of our total body weight is water? Water is our life force. In fact, you could go only a few days without water before your body would start to deteriorate and die. Every day your body uses water for all its internal cellular functions. We lose about 64 ounces of water every day through cellular metabolism and perspiration. Cover your entire arm with a plastic bag and within a few minutes you will get a very visual demonstration of how much water we lose in a day. The eight–glasses–of–water–every day prescription surfaced from the need to replenish the water that is lost every day through cellular respiration. Unfortunately, most people exist on a daily basis in a dehydrated state. Common complaints like headaches, lack of energy, tired and lethargic sensations, injuries, hot flashes and achy joints and muscles have been associated with dehydration. If most people would commit to drinking eight glasses of water every day they would notice a great improvement in their overall health and energy.

Think of it this way: Every tissue, cell, organ and system is composed of water and functions optimally only in the presence of adequate water levels. Degeneration associated with aging will occur at a quicker rate if you are dehydrated. And you can't use thirst to help you determine when you should be drinking water, because as you age your thirst mechanism does not function as well as it should.

My clients who have committed to consuming the right amount of water every day have noticed a huge improvement in their fitness level and body composition. You will, too.

If you are an exerciser, that is another story. In an hour of exercise, you may lose almost two pints of water or more to help dissipate the heat that is being produced. If you exercise, you need to drink those eight glasses a day and, in addition, replenish the water you have lost during your workout. Follow this prescription: Drink water before exercise, during exercise, after exercise and in between!

Take my word for it: water is definitely something that needs to be a priority. Here are two common questions I get from clients regarding water intake:

Every time I commit to drinking more water, I seem to spend all my time running to the washroom. Is there anything I can do about this? In the beginning, your body and its tissues are not accustomed to absorbing this higher level of fluid and will flush it out. Yes, you will be spending a great deal of time in the restroom, but this will not last long. Eventually, your body and its tissues will start to absorb the water and your need to run to the washroom should decrease. Your body will soon adapt to your hydrated state. Your thirst mechanism will also become more efficient; you will find that the more you drink, the thirstier you become. That is a great sign!

Does it have to be water? I suggest that you consume at least eight glasses of good, wholesome, refreshing water every day. Any additional fluids you consume in the form of juice, milk or herbal teas will be a bonus.

Antiaging Nutrition Habit #3

Consume five small meals and snacks throughout the day. See if you recognize yourself in any of the following. You skip breakfast, guzzle coffee all morning and then, practicing great self–control, you eat a tiny lunch. By midafternoon you are starving, so you grab a quick pick–me–up chocolate bar or muffin. By the time you get home you are hungry, irritable, tired and ready for dinner. You stuff yourself at the dinner table and then snack all evening. You go to bed on a full stomach, and next morning the cycle begins again.

This type of eating pattern is common and has your body working against you rather than for you. Many people who do not eat breakfast and consume only a very light lunch are tricked into believing that they are reducing their caloric intake when, in fact, they are setting themselves up for a snacking binge in the late afternoon, followed by an overload at dinner and into the evening. The result is just the opposite of what you intend. Total calories consumed during the day will end up being higher rather than lower! And the scale gives you the bad news that you are gaining weight. This is not what we want to happen as we get older.

The theory is this: Our bodies are not very good at burning calories from a big meal, especially in the evening when all our systems tend to slow down. Many of our evening calories, then, are more likely to be stored as fat. To further complicate matters, eating late at night has been associated with increased episodes of hot flashes and gastrointestinal problems.

Your metabolism, the rate at which you burn calories for internal functions, is like an engine — the more often you give it fuel, the better it works. When you deprive your body of food, even for short periods, your metabolism automatically slows down to preserve energy. A slowed metabolism makes it much more difficult to lose weight and much easier to gain weight. A diet that is not consistent in caloric and nutrient intake will also lead to a more rapid loss of muscle tissue, which we want to avoid at all costs. The good news is that you can get your body to work for you instead of against you. The rule should be that you do not go any longer than four hours during the daytime without eating something.

Think of starting your day by revving your internal engine. This means, regardless of whether you are a "breakfast person" or not, you must develop the habit of having something to eat in the morning. Your momma was right — breakfast is the most important meal of the day — but it does not need to be a five-course meal. A piece of fruit, a bagel, cereal and milk or toast and juice will do the trick. A few hours later, try a small snack such as a piece of fruit or a cup of yogurt. By lunchtime you are not going to have a problem making a healthy, low-fat, low-calorie choice. A half sandwich and salad or bowl of chili or vegetable soup might be an appropriate lunch. A few hours later, in the afternoon, eat another light snack such as a few celery and carrot sticks or crackers and cheese. By the time dinner comes around you will not be ravenous, and you will be less likely to indulge and consume too many calories.

This type of eating pattern keeps your metabolism revved all day, your blood sugar at a healthy level and your energy levels up, and it will help avoid the tendency to overeat at any meal. You'll be a lot more enjoyable to be around, too, because you won't be as irritable as most of us get when we're hungry.

Most of us have been conditioned to believe that dinner should be the largest meal of the day, so changing your eating patterns is not going to be easy. It will not happen overnight. You will probably have to change other old habits, too. If, for example, you snack in the evening while watching TV, you might need to go for a walk in the evening instead. If you find yourself bored in the evening and eating because there is nothing else to do, think about enrolling in an evening course or reading a good book. Breaking habits is very difficult in the beginning, but eventually it will become second nature.

Antiaging Nutrition Habit #4

Reduce Fat Intake. Dietary fat is very easily converted to body fat, so controlling your fat intake is important in controlling the weight gain associated with aging. Limit any food choices that are higher than 30 per cent fat content. Here is an easy formula to determine the fat content of your favorite foods.

1. Read the label to determine the number of grams of fat per serving.

2. Multiply the grams of fat by nine to determine how many fat calories are in the food. (There are nine calories in one gram of fat.)

Breakfast Options:

- Whole-grain cereal or oatmeal with skim milk and fresh fruit or juice
- Egg-white omelette with vegetables
- Toast or bagel with light cream cheese, jam or soy butter, glass of milk, fruit
- Fruit smoothie
- Nonfat yogurt with nonfat granola, fruit

Lunch Options:

- Grilled skinless breast of chicken, tuna or salmon with steamed vegetables or salad
- Salad with grilled chicken and beans. Use vegetables such as dark leafy greens, tomatoes, peppers, carrots, cucumbers and broccoli. Avoid creamy dressings unless they are low-fat — choose a vinaigrette dressing instead.
- Turkey, tuna or grilled chicken sandwich on whole-grain bread, with lettuce and tomato. Use mustard instead of mayonnaise. Complement with cottage cheese.
- Low-fat soup or chili.

3. Read the label to determine the total number of calories in one serving. It's usually listed under "energy."

4. Divide the number of fat calories by the total number of calories. Multiply this by 100 to determine the fat per centage. If the per centage is 30 or less, the food is a low–fat choice.

While reading the labels, also look at the order of ingredients. If fat is listed as one of the first, second or third ingredients, the product is likely to be high in fat and is best avoided. Items such as lard, animal shortening, oils, butterfat, whole–milk solids, shortening and margarine all are fats.

Some obvious foods to avoid are:
- Fried foods — saturated in fat and oil and calories!
- Creams — very high in fat content
- Processed foods such as cakes and cookies and most precooked entrees

Go for wholesome, fresh foods as the staples in your diet. They will always be higher in nutrients and lower in fat. Processed foods should only complement a diet that is rich in fresh fruits, vegetables and whole wheat grains.

While a reduction in fat is usually a good thing, there is a point of diminishing returns and health risks. Fat is the best fuel ever designed! We can make fat out of almost anything we eat and use it for energy. Can you imagine your car doing that? Put in potatoes and the engine miraculously converts them into gas. In go hot dogs and instantly we get gasoline. Fat is an amazing fuel that provides us with a limitless amount of energy. Instead of hating fat and blaming it for all our problems, we should be astounded and respect it for its outstanding capabilities. Certain fatty acids are also necessary for good health, and some fat–soluble vitamins require fat for absorption into the system. Fat also helps to keep us insulated and warm. Elderly persons who have lost weight due to reduced appetite need to consume a moderate amount of dietary fat to maintain a healthy weight.

There is another reason to be less obsessed about reducing fat to super–low levels: fat contributes to feelings of satiety and helps reduce food cravings. While it's true most people don't have to worry about getting too little fat, many who cut a lot of fat from their diets often eat far too much of other "non-fat" foods that are high in calories.

The key is to make sure that your total fat intake is within the accepted guidelines of 20 to 30 per cent of total daily calories. No more than 10 per cent of this should come from saturated fats. The average fat content of most diets

Dinner Options:
- Pasta with low–fat tomato sauce
- Chicken and vegetable stir–fry
- Shrimp, rice and vegetable stir–fry
- Grilled salmon, chicken or tuna with steamed vegetables
- Homemade pizza with light cheese, chicken and vegetables
- Start each dinner with a salad topped with vinaigrette dressing and lots of green, yellow and orange vegetables.

Snack Options:
- Fruit
- Carrot, celery, broccoli or cauliflower
- Low–fat yogurt
- High–protein fruit/nut/grain bar
- Vegetable juice
- Fig bars

is greater than 43 per cent and this, of course, is what is making our society fatter! The major sources of fat in our diets are dairy foods, ice cream, spreads and sauces, so limit your intake of these items.

If you decide to set your fat intake to 25 per cent of total energy, the number of grams of fat you need to consume daily is, depending on your particular circumstances:

- 30 – 50 if you are a woman or a child
- 40 – 60 if you are a man
- 70 if you are a teenager or very active adult
- 80 – 100 if your job requires heavy physical labor or if you are an endurance athlete
- 30 – 40 if your goal is to lose body fat

When deciding to reduce your fat intake, remember that while there are fats that are obvious — the ones you can see, in foods such as butter, margarine, cooking oils and meat — there are also fats hidden in processed foods such as cakes, cookies and potato chips. It is important to limit your intake from both sources.

Unsaturated fats, especially the monounsaturated ones, are considered healthier; they are found in nuts, seeds, vegetable oils and soft margarine products. Saturated fats are found in animal products such as beef, butter, dairy products and lard; they tend to raise blood cholesterol levels, thereby increasing risk of heart disease. Be cautious in consuming coconut or palm oils; these are vegetable oils, but they contain a large amount of saturated fat. You probably have also heard of transfatty acids. These are the end products of a process called hydrogenation, in which vegetable oils are hardened; margarine contains transfatty acids. You should limit your consumption of this type of fat, which can increase the risk of heart disease.

Antiaging Nutrition Habit #5

Reduce salt and sugar intake. By controlling your salt and sugar intake, you can reduce the risk of developing hypertension and adult–onset diabetes. Take away the salt shaker; there is enough salt in most of the foods we eat without our adding more. If you want to boost the taste of certain foods, use salt–free spices such as basil, garlic, oregano or pepper.

When it comes to watching your sugar intake, choose products with a sugar content that is less than 10 per cent of the total carbohydrate content. It's important to avoid items such as cakes, cookies and ice cream. Also limit your intake of no–fat or low–fat products. You are probably thinking, "What? Limit no–fat foods? But aren't they the answer to all my fat–loss prayers?" What do you think makes no–fat products taste so good? Sugar, and lots of it. And what do you think sugar is? A lot of calories! Excess calories, whether from no–fat cookies or full–fat cookies, are going to show up on our hips and thighs and abs. This is why or population continues to get fatter and fatter in spite of the explosion of no–fat products onto the market.

Antiaging Nutrition Habit #6

Avoid caffeine, alcohol, cigarettes and other drugs. These types of drugs will age you quickly. A high intake of caffeine, alcohol and nicotine inhibits the absorption of calcium into bone and speeds up the process of bone loss.

Smoking is associated with a 60 per cent increase in eye damage, an early onset of menopause and an increased risk of cancer and liver and heart disease.

Caffeine is a very powerful drug with very quick, noticeable and measurable effects on the central nervous system, peripheral nervous system and digestive system. In fact, it's used in many prescription and over–the–counter pills. Like other drugs it is habit–forming, and you will find you have to have more and more caffeine to get the same effect. Caffeine makes a lot of people nervous, jittery, tense and stressed. It can often lead to bowel irritation and diarrhea. It is a diuretic that promotes water loss from the body. Treat caffeine as you would alcohol — a little bit once in a while is okay. Moderation is the key. Stick to one or two small cups a day.

Alcohol contributes to high blood pressure and breast cancer, and it damages your liver. Although alcohol is low in fat content, it is very high in empty calories. It also activates an enzyme that takes up fat from our bloodstream and stores it in fat cells. Therefore, any food you consume in combination with alcohol is more likely to end up in a fat–storage depot area like the hips, thighs and abs. Alcohol also lowers our inhibitions, making us more likely to make poorer food choices.

Antiaging Nutrition Habit #7

Control your portion sizes. Here is a very important message: If at the end of the day you have eaten excess calories from any source, you will store these calories as fat. This, of course, will affect the aging process.

Let's say you consume an extra 1,000 carbohydrate calories in the form of

"We can change, slowly and steadily, if we set our will to it."

— ROBERT BENSON

"Some men are born old, and some never seem so. If we keep well and cheerful we are always young, and at last die in youth, even when years would count us old."

— TRYON EDWARDS

plain pasta. It takes about 23 per cent of these calories to break down the dietary carbohydrate and store it as body fat, so 770 of the 1,000 extra carbohydrate calories will be stored as body fat. Now, let's say you consume an extra 1,000 fat calories in the form of creams. It takes about three per cent of these calories to break down the dietary fat and store it as body fat, so 970 of the 1,000 extra fat calories will be stored as body fat.

It is obviously better to have a diet richer in carbohydrates than in fat, because less of the excess will be stored as body fat, but you gain weight whether your diet is low in fat or not. If your diet contains more calories than you expend in a day, you will gain weight regardless of the source of the calories. You must pay attention to your portion sizes no matter what you're eating. We live in a society that is hooked on super–sizing everything from shakes and fries and cookies to muffins and bagels and restaurant entrées. For many of us, it may not be that our food choices are poor but that we are eating too much.

When reducing food intake and portion sizes, do so in the following order:
1. Reduce fat intake
2. Reduce alcohol intake
3. Reduce sugar intake
4. Reduce starches (pasta, breads, rice)

Try eating from a smaller plate or bowl. When eating out, always order the smaller portion size where there's a choice. Split meals with a friend when dining out — for example, order one salad and one entrée between you and share. Always drink a glass of water before any meal.

Pay attention to serving sizes listed on labels. Sometimes what is listed as one serving is unrealistically small, so you may trick yourself into believing you are consuming an amount low in caloric and fat content when, in fact, you are eating four times the listed serving size. For example, a box of macaroni in cheese sauce (not that this would be a particularly healthy choice) might be listed as four servings but most people would find it only enough food for two. When calculating caloric and fat content in such cases multiply the values listed on the label by two to determine whether it's a healthy choice.

Seniors can experience health problems from consuming too few calories, however. For this reason, as we age we should ensure that our total caloric intake for the day does not fall below 1,200 calories.

Antiaging Nutrition Habit #8

Take a multivitamin but don't overuse vitamins, minerals and antioxidants. Is there such a thing as too much of a good thing? There certainly is, and that's why many people who are blindly taking vitamin and mineral supplements are experiencing health complications. Here's a chart to demonstrate some potential side effects of megadoses of certain vitamins and minerals.

Supplement	Claims	Problems from Excess
Vitamin A	Treats certain cancers. Questionable ability to reduce wrinkles and acne.	Liver damage, birth defects, skin irritation.
Beta–carotene	Reduces risk of cancer, heart disease.	Turns skin yellow; worsens liver damage from alcohol.
Vitamin C	Enhances iron absorption. Reduces colds.	Increases free radicals, kidney stones, diarrhea.
Vitamin E	Reduces heart disease risk. Protects against cancer. Enhances immunity. Questionable ability to reduce wrinkles.	Worsens immune disorders (diabetes, etc.) and autoimmune disorders (lupus, etc.).
Fiber	Lowers cholesterol. Lowers risk of colon cancer. Helps control glucose. Questionable ability to lower weight.	Can cause gastrointestinal obstruction; decreases absorption of calcium, zinc, iron.
Omega–3 fatty acids	Lowers cholesterol. Lowers blood pressure. Questionable ability to lower risk of heart disease.	Vitamin A toxicity, increases cholesterol, increases bleeding problems.
Iron	No proof it helps to provide energy.	Promotes diabetes, liver disease, heart disorders; reduces zinc and calcium absorption. Note: Seniors should not take iron supplements unless diagnosed with iron–deficiency anemia.

Supplement	Claims	Problems from Excess
Lecithin	Questionable ability to lower cholesterol. No proof it helps to cure arthritis, improve memory loss, reduce skin problems, gallstones or nervous disorders. No proof it aids weight loss.	Excessive sweating, appetite loss, gastrointestinal distress, excessive salivation, depression, nervous system disorders. Note: The body makes all the lecithin it needs; supplements are not needed.
Phosphorus	Helps build bone.	Stimulates parathyroid glands to draw calcium from bones. The higher the level of phosphorus, the lower the calcium.
Niacin	Lowers cholesterol.	Liver damage, hot flushes, itchy skin, gastrointestinal upset.
Selenium	Reduces risk of cancer in selenium–deficient persons.	In large amounts, severe toxicity, increased risk of cancer, diarrhea, hair/nail loss.

Modified from Herbert, V., & T. Stopler Kasdan. 1994. "Misleading Nutrition Claims and Their Gurus." Nutrition Today 29(3): 28–35 as seen in Kasdan, T. S., 1997. *"A Recipe for Aging"* IDEA Today November/December 1997: 33–41

If you decide to supplement your diet, you should consult with your physician or registered dietitian to ensure you are doing so safely and effectively.

However, it is safe to recommend that you take one multivitamin every day. Choose one that gives close to 100 per cent of the requirements of as many vitamins and minerals as possible.

You may also want to consider taking a calcium–magnesium supplement. The suggested optimal calcium intake is 1,000 milligrams for men, pre-menopausal women, and postmenopausal women taking hormone replacement therapy. For postmenopausal women not taking hormone replacement therapy, 1,500 milligrams of calcium is suggested. Women should consume about 200 milligrams of magnesium, while men need to consume about 400 milligrams of magnesium. Calcium carbonate (ask your pharmacist or doctor) is the most usable form and should be taken with food. Speak with your physician regarding proper dosage and timing of intake. If calcium carbonate causes constipation, calcium citrate may be a better alternative.

I'm sure you've all heard about the much–touted health benefits of antioxidants and the damaging affects of free radicals. One of the theories about aging is that free radicals help cause the process. Free radicals, renegade oxygen molecules, supposedly wreak havoc on DNA structures. An antioxidant is a substance that can donate an electron to a compound, thereby rendering free radicals harmless.

There are three types of antioxidants:

1. Food–based vitamins including A, C and E

2. Phytochemicals, also found in foods and with properties similar to vitamins A, C and E

3. Selenium, an intracellular mineral

What is the right amount of antioxidant consumption? The answer, so far, is highly debatable and the controversy over prescribing adequate but not excessive amounts continues. There is an explosion of compelling and consistent data associating diets rich in fruits and vegetables with a lower cancer risk, which has led physicians and health experts to strongly encourage clients and patients to increase their fruit and vegetable intake. However, the data on using supplements are inconsistent and, moreover, suggest that large doses of supplements may lead to health problems rather than benefits. For this reason, it is wise to consult your physician or nutritionist before taking more than one multivitamin a day.

For vegetarians, it may be necessary to supplement certain vitamins and minerals. For example, vitamin B12 is found only in red meat so if you do not consume red meat, you will need to ensure your diet consists of products that are vitamin B12–fortified, such as cereal, or take supplements. Vegetarians are also candidates for manganese supplementation. Again, talk to your physician.

Antiaging Nutrition Habit #9

Consider hormonal therapy. Many women experiencing the initial stages of menopause decide whether or not they will take hormonal therapy. Estrogen remains the best overall treatment for menopausal women, due to its ability to reduce the rate of bone loss, memory loss and risk of heart disease, as well as to improve sleep and relieve episodes of hot flashes. I'm not pointing you in either direction; see your physician for help in making an educated decision based on your specific health factors.

Here are some of the benefits:

- Helps prevent osteoporosis. Calcium is best used in the presence of estrogen. It is estimated that if all eligible women took this therapy, 50 to 70 per cent of osteoporotic fractures would be prevented.

- Helps reduce hip and spinal compression fractures.

- Reduces risk of cardiovascular disease by 50 per cent (40 per cent of women die from heart disease) because estrogen raises levels of HDL — the "good" cholesterol.

- Increases libido. As you lose estrogen, you also lose androgens.

- Decreases episodes of hot flashes.

- Improves short–term memory. Estrogen supplements may cut the risk of developing Alzheimer's disease by 50 per cent.

- Reduces urinary incontinence.

- Improves sleep patterns.

Here are some of the problems associated with hormonal therapy:

- Increased risk of breast cancer (10 per cent of women die from breast cancer).

- Uterine tumors grow more quickly in the presence of estrogen.

- Contraindicated for individuals suffering from vein and liver disease, and breast or endometrial cancer.

Some women decide against hormone therapy and instead use a diet rich in phytoestrogens as their answer to menopause. To relieve hot flashes and other symptoms they consume large quantities of certain foods — primarily soybean products — that contain estrogen–like compounds. However, many physicians warn against this protocol because the safety and efficacy of these foods have not been studied sufficiently. The intake of phytoestrogens varies according to

> "We have aspects of ourselves hidden deep within, waiting to blossom in our later years…"
>
> — KEN DYCHTWALD

the food sources, and high concentrations may be less safe than an approved pharmaceutical product, especially if progesterone is not provided for endometrial protection as would routinely be done with hormonal therapy.

Other women take natural herbal remedies, but many physicians are also cautious about these because the industry is unregulated and more research is required to substantiate claims.

New research is coming to the forefront on these issues every day, so it is critical that you consult your physician regarding alternative therapies to manage menopause. Regularly review the latest findings to learn how they may affect your decision.

Finally, you know what they say: you are what you eat. If you are serious about slowing down the rate at which you're aging, you must adhere to the suggestions in this strategy. Looking good and feeling great is definitely within your reach.

"To me, old age is always 15 years older than I am ..."

— BERNARD M. BARUCH

Mind Body Relaxation Training & Stress Management Techniques

Let's face it, in our time people are running from appointment to appointment, deadline to deadline. You have two dozen e–mails and nine voice messages waiting to be answered. Your cell phone is ringing again. You're a half hour late for your next appointment. You were up late last night working on a project. You haven't called your best friend in more than a week. You haven't spent "quality time" with your kids since the weekend. Whatever happened to the days when you actually got home at around 5:30 p.m., had dinner with your family and sat on the front porch talking with your neighbors? Today, people count themselves fortunate if they get home by 8 or 9 p.m. The following extract from a poem, written and emailed by a student at Columbine High School, sums it all up:

> The paradox of our time in history is that we have taller buildings, but shorter tempers; wider freeways, but narrower viewpoints; we spend more, but have less; we buy more, but enjoy it less.
>
> We have bigger houses and smaller families; more conveniences, but less time; we have more degrees, but less sense; more knowledge, but less judgment; more experts, but more problems; more medicine, but less wellness.
>
> We have multiplied our possessions, but reduced our values. We talk too much, love too seldom and hate too often. We've learned how to make a living, but not a life. We've added years to life, but not life to years. We've been all the way to the moon and back, but have trouble crossing the street to meet the new neighbour.
>
> These are the days of two incomes, but more divorce; of fancier houses, but broken homes. It is a time when there is much in the shop window and nothing in the stockroom; a time when technology can bring this letter to you, and a time when you can choose whether to make a difference or just hit delete.
>
> It's time.

Pretty impactful, isn't it? Raises a lot of questions, doesn't it? Much of the stress we experience may be self–imposed because we are trying to achieve something we believe will bring us happiness. We may believe that going faster is the way to get more time. We may be overwhelmed by how much we have to get done, so speed up to try to accomplish more. Many of us often cut down on "extras" such as exercise, sleep and seeing family and friends so that

"Growing old should
be a rich summation
of experience, not
a decay ..."

— CONSTANCE WARREN

we have more time to get things done. No wonder most of our society is feeling so empty and turning to alcohol, drugs, overeating or cigarettes. It reminds me so much of Orson Welles's classic film *Citizen Kane*. If you remember the story, it was about a young boy whose mother came into some money and sent him away to the best schools. He grew up to be one of the wealthiest, most influential men on the planet. He had everything money could buy. But he also had two failed marriages, no solid friendships and lots of enemies. On his deathbed, he whispers one word — "Rosebud" — the name of the sled he used to play with when he lived with his mom. The camera fades away with a clip of his estate and all his possessions being burned. In that instant the message is clear. He spent his entire life trying to make money to collect the things that all were destroyed in the end. And the only happy memory he had when he died was not of the money or the things or his business or his multimillion dollar estate. It was that of playing in the snow when he was a young child — when life seemed simpler.

We can take the message at heart and ask ourselves, do we have our priorities in order? Are we doing the things we want to be doing? Why do we let little things get to us? Successful stress management happens first by taking a different perspective on our lives and adjusting our attitudes and actions accordingly.

Too many of us put our jobs first and squeeze everything else into the time that's left. We have things to do, people to see and much to accomplish. Sixty–one per cent of American workers say they never have enough time to get everything down. Sixty–five per cent say their job requires them to work very fast. Fifty–six per cent say they have to work on too many tasks at the same time. And if you examine the work habits and health of senior executives who work on average 11.9 hours per day, it's no wonder 40 per cent are obese, 73 per cent are not physically active, and 75 per cent have two or more risk indicators for cardiovascular disease.

All you need is a wake–up call, and I hope this it. Life is too short to be worrying about the past or the future or spending all your time at the office. Perhaps you're going to have to make some major changes in your life to allow time for the things that are most important to you. You might need to set a goal of how many dinners per week you'll eat with your family. You may decide to not work on the weekends or choose at least Saturday or Sunday to have a full day off. You may have to say "no" to more work demands, turn down additional tasks, projects or promotions if they will undermine your quality of life or hurt your relationships. You may have to choose one night per week as a "date night" with your spouse or to go out with your friends. Make today the day you start to put your life back in balance.

So where do you start? In addition to a change of attitude, if there are things that help you to reduce your stress levels and increase your energy, do them. Some people enjoy bubble baths; others like to read or get a massage. Deep, slow breathing may help you. Shopping may do the trick. Others like to go for a walk or call a good friend or their parents. Some people enroll in a tai chi or meditation class. Do what it takes to help you achieve a relaxed, calm state. Your health will improve noticeably.

Mind/Body Programs:

We can't really expect our bodies to cooperate if we don't treat them well. We can't expect to take care of others if we don't first establish a priority of taking care of our own health. These realizations, along with rising health–care costs and the aging of health–conscious baby boomers, are primary reasons for the increasing popularity of mind/body disciplines such as yoga, tai chi, meditation and Pilates–based programs.

IDEA, the International Health and Fitness Organization, reports that a growing body of scientific evidence supports mindful exercise as a significant means of favorably altering various aspects of health. Scientific research on yoga has been enormous (well over 2,000 studies) since the first research began in the 1920s, and since 1985 approximately 1,500 research abstracts have been published on chi kung (also known as qi gong) and tai chi. Ralph LaForge, a physician specializing in the benefits of mind/body exercise, sums up the benefits:

Meditation and mindful exercise have been credited with [being] effective at complementing existing stress and anger management programs; reducing the medical and economical costs of psychological distress; improving muscular strength, flexibility, balance and coordination; reducing falls in the elderly; improving glucose tolerance; increasing heart–rate variability and cardiac parasympathetic tone; improving cardiac reactivity related to work strain; reducing responsiveness to stress hormones; increasing self–awareness and personal empowerment; decreasing anxiety and neuroticism; decreasing trait anxiety; decreasing pain and pain sensitization; reducing blood pressure; improving lipid profile; improving bone mineral density; improving pulmonary function; improving cardiorespiratory fitness; decreasing mortality and/or clinical events associated with cardiovascular disease, and decreasing ischemic response to exercise.

Wow, that's a long list of benefits!

In the Flexibility Training section, we reviewed a number of yogic poses that I encourage you to practice regularly or alternatively, purchase a Pilates video or enroll in a tai chi class.

Here are some other techniques to help you slow down.

Breathing

The first thing you do when you are born is breathe, and it's the last thing you'll do when you exit. Oxygen is the most vital nutrient for our bodies and is essential for all of our organs and tissues. If we don't get enough of it, the result is mental sluggishness, negative thoughts, depression and various other health concerns. The act of breathing seems pretty simple and mindless, but most of us will find when we think about it that our breath is very shallow and quick and we often hold it. Think about how your breathing changes if you're angry, sad, stressed or afraid.

By practicing deep breathing you can expect:

- Improved quality in the blood, due to its increased oxygenation in the lungs.

- Increased digestion and assimilation of food. The digestive organs such as the stomach receive more oxygen and hence operate more efficiently.

- Improved health in the nervous system, including the brain, spinal cord and nerve centers. This in turn improves your overall health, as the nervous system communicates with all parts of the body.

- Rejuvenated skin.

- Stimulated blood circulation as the movements of the diaphragm during deep breathing massage the abdominal organs.

- Healthier and more powerful lungs.

- Reduced workload for the heart. This results in a stronger, more efficient heart, reduced blood pressure and less heart disease.

- Relaxation of the mind and body. Deep breathing causes a reflex relaxation of the mind. In addition, oxygenation of the brain tends to normalize brain function, reducing excessive anxiety levels.

Kolber, P., B.R.E.A.T.H., IDEA World Fitness Summit, Anaheim, CA 2000

When you're in need of a mental break, try the following exercises:

Deep Breathing

INHALING

1. Push your stomach forward as you breathe in through your nose.

2. Push your ribs sideways while still breathing in. Your stomach will automatically go inward slightly.

3. Lift your chest and collarbone while still breathing in.

EXHALING

1. Allow your collarbone, chest and ribs to relax. The air will go out automatically.

2. When all the air seems to be out, push your stomach in slightly to expel any remaining air.

Diaphragmatic Breathing

1. Lie down on a rug or blanket, your legs straight and slightly apart, toes pointed comfortably outward, arms at your sides, not touching your body and palms up, eyes closed.

2. Bring your attention to your breathing and place your hand on the spot that seems to rise and fall most as you breathe.

3. Gently place both of your hands on your abdomen and become aware of your breathing.

4. Breathe through your nose.

5. As you breathe in, allow the abdomen to expand without forcing or arching the back.

6. Exhale, emptying the abdomen completely.

"It is magnificent to grow old, if one keeps young ..."

— HARRY E. FOSDICK

Alternate Nostril Breathing

1. Sit in a comfortable position, with good posture.

2. Close your right nostril with your right thumb.

3. Inhale slowly and soundlessly through your left nostril.

4. Immediately close the left nostril with your right ring finger and little finger. At the same time, remove your thumb from the right nostril.

5. Exhale slowly and soundlessly through your right nostril.

6. Inhale through your right nostril.

7. Close your right nostril with your thumb and open your left nostril.

8. Exhale through your left nostril.

9. Inhale through your left nostril.

   Repeat the cycle.

"Fun, frivolity, merriment are the things essential to the normal mind, as rain is necessary to the flowers ..."

— FRED VAN AMBURGH

Breath of Fire

1. Kneel on the floor or sit in a comfortable position.

2. Keep your back straight, with shoulders back and down. Place your hands on your abdomen.

3. Take a deep breath. Round your lips and begin to blow the breath out through your mouth by strongly contracting your abdominal wall.

4. As you release your abdomen, the breath will be drawn in.

5. Each exhalation should be directed and careful. The inhalation will take care of itself.

Contract/Relax

Take a moment to contract and tense all the muscles in your body. Immediately relax them. Repeat this three to five times. You can do this drill with your entire body all at once, or body part by body part.

Take a Minutes Vacation

Stop what you're doing. Close your eyes. Take a few deep breaths. Imagine a scene from nature that relaxes and calms you. Perhaps take yourself to a deserted island, to the top of a mountain or to an ocean beach.

Here and Now

Stop what you're doing. Close your eyes. Take a few deep breaths. Become aware of your environment. What do you hear? What do you smell? What do you feel? Open your eyes. What do you see?

> There is always something to laugh about every day, even if it is only about yourself."
>
> — FRED VAN AMBURGH

Laugh

Having a sense of humor affects us on several levels. From a physiological standpoint, laughter stimulates many of the same positive physiological changes we experience after exercise: deeper breathing, lower heart rate, decreased blood pressure and an influx of endorphins. On a psychological level, humor creates a sense of lightheartedness and play.

How can you incorporate humor into your life?

- Nourish your comic spirit by taking in a steady diet of funny movies and comedians.

- Collect cartoons and include them on memos, agendas or presentations at work and on the fridge at home.

- When planning a meeting at work, schedule something fun on the agenda.

- Lose any pessimism in your spirit.

- Get amusing screen savers for your computer.

- Exchange good, tasteful jokes or other funny material via e-mail.

- Have a party.

- Surround yourself with fun, lively people.

- Laugh a minimum of 20 times per day.

McLaughlin, P., CatchFire: A 7–Step Program to Ignite Energy, Defuse Stress, and Power Boost Your Performance. – A FitnessAge Corporate Program.

Prayer

Prayer and a belief in God has been crucial to a sense of peace and well–being since the beginning of time, and recently, science is proving that prayer works. Scientists are opening theirs minds to the healing powers of faith. A study by Dr. Chandrakant Shah, a professor of public health sciences at the University of Toronto Faculty of Medicine, showed that people who are spiritual tend to live longer. It makes sense — someone who follows God's will generally tends to be more forgiving, loving and kind, less likely to fall prey to the temptations of alcohol and drugs and more likely to be at peace versus being stressed. In hospitals, medical studies have shown that patients who pray before and after surgery recover faster than their non–praying peers. Even God tells us in Proverbs 3: 1–8

> *My son, do not forget my law,*
> *But let your heart keep my commands;*
> *For length of days and long life*
> *And peace they will add to you.*
> *Let not mercy and truth forsake you;*
> *Bind them around your neck,*
> *Write them on the tablet of your heart,*
> *And so find favor and high esteem*
> *In the sight of God and man.*
> *Trust in the Lord with all your heart,*
> *And lean not on your own understanding;*
> *In all your ways acknowledge Him,*
> *And He shall direct your paths.*
> *Do not be wise in your own eyes;*
> *Fear the Lord and depart from evil.*
> *It will be health to your flesh,*
> *And strength to your bones.*

Wow, God promises us quite a few blessings if we trust in him — peace, a long life, health and strength. So how do you pray correctly? Most people are shocked to learn that to have a relationship with God doesn't require going to church or a synagogue every week. In fact, never once does God command that we must attend church to be closer to him. Instead, he tells believers the temple of God is within us (2 Corinthians 5:16b). In John 4: 1–26, Jesus shows us that God is not as concerned with where we pray or worship but how we pray.

So you can draw close to God right now; you can do it in your office or while you're hiking on top of a beautiful mountain. You can do it today — you don't have to wait until Saturday or Sunday. You don't have to shut your eyes, or bring your hands into prayer position or get down onto your knees to have a conversation with God. Just start talking to Him. Ask Him to guide you in your life. Ask for His will in your life. Change your mind. Although we've talked a lot about the importance of exercise and healthy eating, "The Kingdom of God is not eating and drinking but righteousness, peace and joy in the Holy Spirit." (Romans 14:17). And this peace and joy and happiness are the most sought after commodities in our society today. God promises us that if we seek, we will find, and if we knock, the door will be opened. (Matthew 6:7–8).

Remember this:

Fitness is not only physical health but mental and spiritual health as well.

Pelvic Floor Exercises

An inability to control urine flow as we age can be a socially embarrassing problem, but it can be managed. Stress incontinence — the loss of urine when you cough, sneeze, laugh or jump — is generally a result of a weakening of the pelvic floor muscles. It makes sense that if you strengthen those particular muscles you'll reduce the chances of having to endure regular awkward, episodes.

A plan of action can start immediately with Kegel exercises. Named for inventor and American physician A. H. Kegel, these involve contracting and releasing muscles to improve bladder control.

The correct way to perform a Kegel is as follows. Imagine that you are going to the bathroom; imagine that you have interrupted the flow of urine. The muscles you use to stop the flow are your pelvic floor muscles and these are the ones you want to strengthen. You shouldn't condition the muscles while actually going to the bathroom, because many therapists have cautioned that this type of disruption can lead to infections. However, now that you know what the sensation is you can regularly do Kegel exercises to condition these muscles and apply that control when you need it.

There are two protocols for pelvic floor exercises, one for each of the two major types of incontinence: stress and endurance incontinence. Consult your physician or physical therapist; a biofeedback examination can determine which you have. If you have both conditions, or have neither and just want to take a preventive approach, follow both protocols.

For stress incontinence, perform 10 reps of "quick flicks" — short, one- to two- second contractions with two- to four-second rests in between. Start with one session of 10 reps, three times per week. Build up to three sessions of 10 reps, three times per week. For endurance incontinence (trouble holding), contract your pelvic floor muscles for 10 seconds, then relax for 20 seconds. For this protocol, the rest period should always be twice as long as the active period to ensure adequate muscle recovery. Start with 10 reps, four to five times per week. Build to a 20–second contraction, with a 40–second rest, four to five times per week. Many people think they are holding firmly for the full length of the contraction, but biofeedback shows an initial peak contraction followed by a rapid decline. To prevent this, draw the muscles upward tightly, then, throughout the contraction, repeatedly tighten, tighten, tighten, about once per second.

"Do not be afraid to demand great things of yourself. Powers which you never dreamed you possessed will leap to your assistance…"

— ORISON S. MARDEN

With pelvic floor exercising, some studies show detraining after three months of overtraining. If this occurs, cut back your program to about 50 percent of effort and continue at this rate until retraining occurs. Then slowly rebuild.

Pelvic floor muscles are co–contractors with other muscles such as abs (especially rectus and transverse abs), glutes and the respiratory diaphragm. If you engage the pelvic floor muscles when training these other muscles, you'll get more power out of latter.

If doing resistance training that involves holding the breath during lifting or other maximal efforts, it's best to engage the pelvic floor muscles. Otherwise, intraabdominal pressure will create strain on them.

Pelvic floor muscles (along with transverse abdominus) play an important part in malalignment of the spine and sacrum, so engage them when doing back exercises, especially for the lower back.

Many therapists are now suggesting that exercisers contract their pelvic floor muscles before they initiate any type of exercise. For example, if you're about to perform an overhead shoulder press, start by contracting your abdominals, lifting your chest up and out and your shoulders back and contracting your pelvic floor muscles. Then you can start the exercise. Kegels are beneficial to both men and women, but since women are at a higher risk for stress incontinence these exercises are a must for them.

Sexual Intercourse

We've already discussed briefly some of the problems that can occur with your intimate life as you age. As with anything else, if you don't use it, you lose it! Research supports the view that regular sexual intercourse is the key to preventing some of the changes in our sexual organs as we age. In fact, sexual intercourse three times per month is the major contributing factor in helping to prevent the thinning and drying of the vaginal wall. It promotes blood flow to the vaginal wall and keeps tissues thick, soft and lubricated.

You heard it here first: Do your weights twice a week, cardio three to five times per week and enjoy sex with your spouse about once a week.

If you've already experienced significant drying and thinning and sexual intercourse is painful, march down to your local drugstore and pick up some vaginal lubricant. This will help you get through the initial stages. Also request from your spouse a little longer foreplay to help initiate the secretion of fluids.

"Anyone who keeps the ability to see beauty never grows old."

— FRANZ KAFKA

Sun Protection

Thanks in large part to our desire for the "perfect" tan, we are spending more time in the sun (and in tanning booths) than our skin can tolerate. As a result skin cancer, once common mainly among those people who had to work in the sun, is occurring with alarming frequency. Severe sunburning during childhood and chronic sun exposure during adolescence and younger adulthood are thought to be responsible for contributing to this increase in skin cancer.

Things don't get any better as we get older. Our skin loses some of its natural suppleness, and many of us — men especially — through baldness and thinning hair find that we are exposing sensitive skin. It may also be in our middle years that bad sunning habits of our youth begin to catch up with us.

The key to successful treatment of skin cancer lies in early detection. In the case of basal or squamous cell cancer, the most common forms of skin cancer, the development of a pale, waxlike, pearly nodule or red scaly patch may be the first symptom. For others, skin cancer may be reflected in the changing configuration of an already existing skin mole. If such a change is noted, a physician should be consulted. Melanomas usually begin as a small, molelike growth that grows progressively in size, changes color, ulcerates, and bleeds easily. For use in detecting these melanomas, the American Cancer Society recommends the following alert guidelines:

A is for asymmetry.

B is for border irregularity.

C is for color change.

D is for a diameter greater than six millimeters (0.24 inches).

Most of us experience some changes in skin pigmentation as we age, so–called "liver spots" among them. Most of these are benign, but if you have any concerns about new or unusual spots on your skin consult your physician.

Fortunately, when skin cancer is detected various treatment methods can be used. Surgery, radiation and tissue destruction by heat or by freezing are frequently combined to achieve an almost 100 percent cure rate. For the more serious and difficult–to–cure melanomas, more extensive surgery will be required to make certain that the cancerous cells and surrounding lymph nodes have been removed.

"There is no finer or more fitting way to spend time during the evening years of life than turning the mind toward reflection and then stilling it in the silence..."

— PAUL BRUNTON

Nothing ages our skin more quickly than the sun. So be sun smart and always wear sunscreen — even in the winter — on exposed areas. Wear sunglasses and hats to block out the harmful rays and avoid long exposure to the sun during the midday hours, when the most damaging ultraviolet radiation is at its peak.

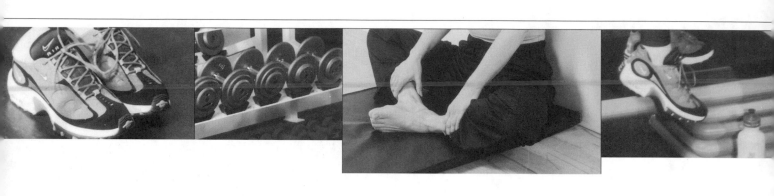

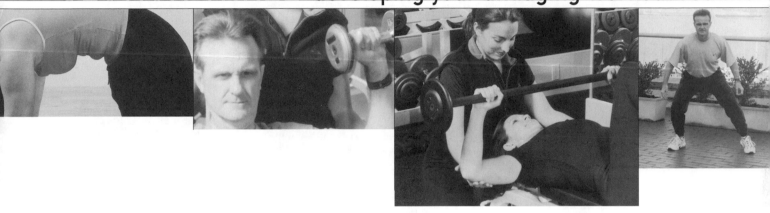

It's now time to design your sample weekly fitness program. Decide on which days you'll exercise and on which you'll rest. Decide which activities you'll do on each day and for how long.

Remember, you need three to five cardio workouts of varying intensity and duration. You should ensure you include a bit of interval, agility and balance training within your routine. You also need two muscle-conditioning workouts that will involve exercises for your lower body, upper body and torso. Ensure you save lots of time to stretch and relax. Oh, yeah, and don't forget your Kegels and you-know-what once a week.

Sample Personal Exercise Program

Mon	Tues	Wed	Thurs	Fri	Sat	Sun
AM	**AM**	**AM**	**AM**	Rest	**AM**	**AM**
45 minute walk + abdominal stabilization exercises + yoga stretches	upper and lower body resistance training program + wall stretches	30 minute walk + abdominal stabilization exercises + yoga stretches	upper and lower body resistance training program + wall stretches		1-hour bike ride + agility and balance exercises + wall stretches	20-minute run/walk (4 min. walking, 1 min. running) x 4 + yoga stretches
PM	**PM**	**PM**	**PM**			
End-of-day postural stretches, breathing exercises	End-of-day postural stretches, breathing exercises	End-of-day postural stretches, breathing exercises	End-of-day postural stretches, breathing exercises			

Your Ideal Personal Exercise Program

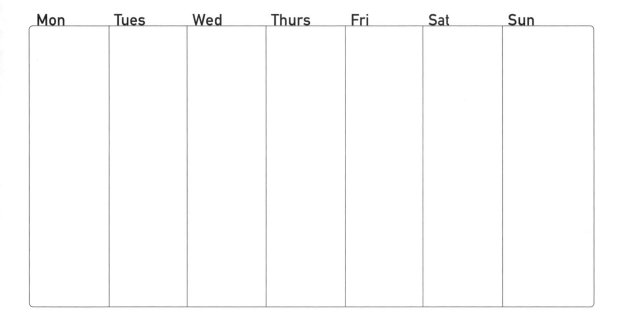

Mon	Tues	Wed	Thurs	Fri	Sat	Sun

When designing your program, it is imperative that you set an ideal and a maintenance goal. For example, your ideal cardiovascular goal may be five workouts per week, but your minimal goal will take into consideration weeks when you are really busy at work, not feeling so hot or away on holiday. This will prevent you from getting off track and backsliding. This maintenance goal will be the minimal exercise you will commit to, even if life is rough. This will ensure that you maintain your level of fitness. Generally, if you manage to do one good, high–intensity cardio– and muscle–conditioning workout in a week when things are crazy you will maintain your fitness, provided you maintain your program during weeks in which events cut you more slack. Take the time now to record your ideal exercise goal and your maintenance exercise goal.

Ideal Goal _____ **Maintenance Goal** _____

I suggest you review your program design every four to eight weeks. Make some changes. Introduce a new activity. Learn some new exercises. Change the order and sequencing of your workout days; this is where the investment in seeing a personal fitness trainer for a couple sessions will pay off. Don't make the mistake of designing one program and relying on it for improved health and fitness for years to come. Regular change, a minimum of every two months, is fundamental to ongoing progress.

Should You Work Out if You're Not Feeling Well?

Whether to work out while unwell concerns many exercisers. Although more research is needed, the general guideline is that if you have symptoms of a common cold, with no fever and all symptoms above the neck, moderate exercise such as walking should be okay. However, if your symptoms include fever, extreme tiredness, muscle aches or swollen lymph glands you should refrain from exercise until you get better. When you do start exercising again, progress slowly and gently. Even if you do have to take a week or two off because you're feeling under the weather, it really won't make that much difference to your overall fitness level if you're consistent with your program the rest of the time.

If you get sick often, why? Is there something you can do about it? Once you've been exposed to a virus, the likelihood of your getting sick depends on a number of factors, including advancing age, whether you smoke, high levels of stress, poor nutrition and lack of sleep. Exercisers frequently report that they experience less sickness than their sedentary peers. (The American Council on Exercise reports that 61 per cent of 700 recreational runners studied had fewer colds after they began running, while only four per cent reported the frequency had increased.) During moderate exercise, various immune cells circulate through the body more quickly and are better able to kill bacteria and viruses. So every time you go for a brisk walk your immune system receives a boost that could increase your chances of fighting off respiratory infections.

Exercise won't guarantee that you won't get sick. In fact, sometimes too much exercise can put you at greater risk of developing a virus. A high per centage of marathoners and triathletes get sick immediately after a big event. The theory is that too much exercise may suppress the immune system and make you more susceptible to catching viruses.

Here are some general tips to reduce your odds of getting sick.

Eat well: The immune system depends on many vitamins, minerals and sufficient caloric intake for optimal functioning. Make sure you consume plenty of fruits, vegetables and grain products and drink a minimum of eight glasses of water per day.

Get lots of sleep: The American Council on Exercise reports that major sleep disruption (three hours less than normal) has been linked to immune system suppression.

Exercise: Include moderate levels of exercise in your weekly schedule to ensure your immune system receives a regular boost.

Avoid overtraining: Space vigorous workouts and race events as far apart as possible. Allow for adequate recovery periods and rest days.

Your View from Here

When a fit and healthy 19-year-old throws a ball, then sprints across the lawn to retrieve it, she is the picture of a perfectly tuned machine. Neurons fire rapidly, telling muscles to contract and release; lungs take in oxygen almost without effort, while a strong heart pumps oxygen-rich blood through supple arteries.

What happens to that 19-year-old's body 10 years later, 20 years later, 30 years and more, later if she, like so many of us, gives up chasing balls and begins leading a largely sedentary life? She loses muscle. She loses strength. She is not able to walk up stairs, let alone sprint across the lawn. Her lungs become less adept at taking in oxygen. Her heart weakens. Her bones thin. Her body fat increases, and she tires at the least exertion. She becomes the picture of frail old age.

Is this inevitable? We now know that it's not. Sure, there's not much you can do to stop the graying hair and the wrinkles, but scientists have found the true fountain of youth. It's called exercise, and it can stave off many of the physical changes commonly attributed to aging. A little bit of cardiovascular conditioning, muscle training and good nutrition can preserve muscle tissue, strength, bone density, heart health, energy levels and functional performance. There is no magic pill or drug that can do this for you. Putting one foot in front of the other, making your muscles and heart and lungs work is the key. If you don't use it, you lose it. So start using it and not only will you not lose it, you may be surprised at how much you actually gain!

Good luck and stay fit — physically, mentally and spiritually!

"Be not afraid of growing slowly; be afraid of standing still."

— CHINESE PROVERB

Sherri McMillan, M.Sc., B.H.K., an exercise physiologist, has her bachelor's and master's degrees in exercise science. With her husband, Alex, she is the co-owner of NorthWest Personal Training and Fitness Education in Vancouver, Washington, where she acts as a consultant, presenter, personal trainer and fitness instructor. She has been honored with the inaugural IDEA International Personal Trainer of the Year and the CanFitPro Canadian Fitness Presenter of the Year awards. As Sherri Kwasnicki she authored *Go For Fit: The Winning Way to Fat Loss* (also published by Raincoast Books). She is a featured fitness columnist for various newspapers, magazines and journals including the *Province* newspaper in Vancouver, British Columbia, and *Chatelaine* and *Shape* magazines. She is one of North America's most well–respected fitness leaders and is regularly sought after as an international presenter and lecturer at, among others, IDEA, IHRSA and CanFitPro fitness conferences. A Nike– and PowerBar–sponsored fitness athlete, she loves to hike, run, cycle, swim, in–line skate, rock climb and snowboard in her spare time.

If you have any questions or comments for the author, you can forward them to: Raincoast Books, attention: Sherri McMillan.

Glossary

abdominals (abs): The stomach muscles.

abductors: The outer thigh muscles.

adductors: The inner thigh muscles.

aerobic exercise: Exercise that involves the use of large muscle groups rhythmically and continuously, and elevating the heart rate and breathing for a sustained period. It can be done comfortably for a period of 20 minutes or more. Examples include jogging, walking, cyclying, swimming and fitness classes.

anaerobic exercise: Exercise done at a much higher intensity level than aerobic exercise and for a much shorter duration. It can be done for a period of 30 seconds to two minutes. Examples include resistance and weight training.

anterior deltoids: The front shoulder muscles.

antioxidant: A substance that prevents or slows the breakdown of another substance through the process of oxidation. In the body, antioxidants act by scavenging the naturally occurring but potentially damaging free radicals (chemicals that occur within the body that can cause irreversible damage to cells). The body produces its own antioxidants such as the enzyme superoxide dismutase and other nutrients such as beta-carotene, vitamin C, vitamin E and selenium to keep the number of free radicals in balance. Stress, aging, and environmental sources such as polluted air and cigarette smoke can increase the number of free radicals in the body that can damage healthy DNA.

endurance incontinence: A dysfunction resulting in difficulty controlling movements of the bladder or bowels or both.

free radicals: A molecule or atom that contains an unpaired electron but is neither positively nor negatively charged. Free radicals are usually highly reactive and unstable and have been linked to changes that accompany aging and disease processes that lead to cancer, heart disease and stroke.

gluteals (glutes): Any of the three muscles in each buttock.

hamstrings: The muscles on the back of the thighs.

kyphotic: Hunched back posture caused by excessive curvature of the spine.

latissimus dorsi (lats): The muscles in the lower back.

lunge: An exercise that involves a forward movement and bending of the front leg at the knee while keeping the back leg straight. It works the entire lower body.

medial deltoids: The middle shoulder muscles.

pectorals: The chest muscles.

pilates: A technique that involves strengthening and lengthening muscles. The emphasis of this technique is on core stabilization and training.

quadriceps: The front thigh muscles.

rectus abs: The abdominal muscle that is responsible for the "six-pack" look.

reps, repetitions: The number of times an exercise is performed without stopping.

rhomboids: The back muscle that pulls the shoulder blades together.

set: The number of times a complete series of repetitions is performed. For example, two sets of 10 reps.

squats: An exercise that involves bending at both knees and lowering the torso in a sitting position. The squat conditions the entire lower body.

stress incontinence: A dysfunction resulting in a loss of urine when coughing, laughing, sneezing, jumping or participating in high-impact activities.

tibialis: The shin muscles.

transverse abs: The abdominal muscle that is responsible for pulling the abdominal cavity inwards.

triceps: The large muscle at the back of the upper arm.

Index